The Alkalizing Diet

The Alkalizing Diet

Your Life Is in the Balance

Istvan Fazekas

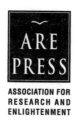

ASSOCIATION FOR
RESEARCH AND
ENLIGHTENMENT

A.R.E. Press • Virginia Beach • Virginia

A.R.E. Press
215 67th Street
Virginia Beach, VA 23451–2061

Library of Congress Cataloguing–in–Publication Data
Fazekas, Istvan, 1964–
    The alkalizing diet : your life is in the balance / by Istvan Fazekas.
      p.   cm.
    ISBN 0-87604-510-7 (trade pbk.)
    1. Nutrition. 2. Food combining. 3. Acid–base equilibrium. 4. Cayce, Edgar, 1877–1945. I. Title.
    RA784.F39 2005
    613.2—dc22

                                        2005013341

Disclaimer

The information in this book is not intended to replace medical advice. You should consult your physician regarding any general or specific physical symptoms. The author and publisher disclaim any responsibility for adverse effects resulting from information in this book.

Cover design by Richard Boyle

Contents

Introduction

AMERICANS SHOULD BE THE HEALTHIEST PEOPLE ON THE PLANET. WE spend the most money per capita on health care and have the most medical technology at our disposal of any industrialized nation. But we are not—not really. We are getting more obese, and the risk of resultant pathologies because of our expanding frames is also increasing. A January 2002 Harris poll[i] states the following:

> Fully 33% [of Americans] are now 20% overweight, a reasonable measure of obesity, compared to 15% in 1983, 16% in 1990, and 22% in 1995. In other words, **obesity has more than doubled from less than one-sixth of the population eighteen years ago to one-third today.** [Author's emphasis]

The idea of one–third of 293 million people being obese—about 98 million Americans—is a startling statistic.[ii] Is our ever–growing weight problem the main cause of our nation's health concern? It is our overall lifestyle, with diet being the number two factor right behind the nefarious nicotine nemesis.

According to the Centers for Disease Control, in 2000 the most common actual causes of death in the United States were tobacco use (435,000), poor diet and physical inactivity (400,000), alcohol consumption (85,000), microbial agents (e.g., influenza and pneumonia, 75,000), toxic agents (e.g., pollutants and asbestos, 55,000), motor vehicle accidents (43,000), firearms (29,000), sexual behavior (20,000), and illicit use of drugs (17,000).[iii]

Almost a million people a year die as a direct result of poor diet, lack of physical activity, smoking, and excessive drinking! (See Figure 1.) Those statistics are likely quite conservative. We have a skyrocketing obesity rate and appear to be victims of our own advancements in comfort and convenience. When health problems are the result, we rely exceedingly on technology to aid us in our time of disease. Often at the expense of common sense, to create the perception of health, we defy the laws of wellness for the quick fix. As a humorous Billy Crystal character from a popular Saturday night comedy show used to say, "It is much better to look good than to feel good, dahling." This may be the new national motto.

This is from the Centers for Disease Control (CDC):[iv]

Figure 1. Most common causes of death in the United States, 1999*

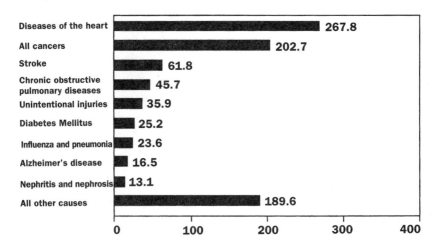

*Rates are age adjusted to 2000 total U.S. population.

Not only are the older generations falling into (or never crawling out of) bad habits, but we have a whole new generation of Americans who see the world of health within very inadequate parameters. The primary concern is that we are breeding an entire generation of youth who are so suspicious or ignorant of the healing power of the natural world that fresh fruits and vegetables will appear as archaic to them as muzzle-loaders and ball bearings appear to the modern soldier.

True confession #2767:
The Orange and the Cheerleader

I was once teaching a class about fascia, the pervasive connective tissue of the body that covers all major anatomical structures, from muscles to bones, tendons to organs. A teaching analogy that I use is an orange. The basic structure of an orange has the pith, which we can use to represent the body's superficial fascia, the connective tissue underneath your skin. The individual orange slices represent each muscle and its own covering. Each pocket within an orange slice represents a distinct structure—that is, muscle cells, nerves, and so forth. From there I introduce the fascinating connective tissue networks, from macro to micro.

During this particular class, a young girl recently out of high school, the captain of her cheerleading team, raised her hand. "What do you mean?" she asked with a look of bewilderment. I explained that the orange represents the way the body has wrappings around its various layers. "I am still confused," she persisted with a tilt of the head, reminiscent of Nipper the dog staring into the old Victrola. "Okay," I gestured toward her and began redrawing my Picasso orange on the white board. "You know when you peel an orange . . . " She stopped me in mid-sentence. "I really don't know what an orange's inside looks like," she sincerely confessed. At first I thought this was a joke of some sort, so I played along. "Come on, you know that orange-colored fruit that comes at the end of the meal at the Chinese restaurant, sometime between the egg fu yung and the fortune cookie." I realized that she was earnest in her appeal as she stated, "I have never seen the inside of an orange. My dad just buys Sunny Delight. I know they have pictures of oranges on the carton, but I've never peeled one." After further exploring this enigma, I came to understand that she also lacked first-hand knowledge of lemons, limes, grapefruit, and apples—the whole distance along the produce bin at the local supermarket.

She was eighteen years old and had never eaten a raw orange or, it appeared, any raw fruit! Cranking my jaw up from the classroom carpet like Wylie E. Coyote, it hit me that I was communicating with a very different generation. This is a generation to whom juice is grown in cartons, derived from some mysterious thing that can only be understood as an advertisement, not an experience in nature. For some in the new generation, it appears that oranges and their mysterious juice are fabricated by scientists at the Sunny Delight factory.

How many people are in the same situation as this young girl? How many adults go months, even years, without seeing raw fruits or fresh vegetables at a meal or having the experience of growing their own? I believe that people being out of touch with growing their own herbs and produce is a key cause of poor health—physical and spiritual. We are losing our contact with the natural world and the spirit of the plant. If you do not connect with the spirit of something, it becomes very difficult, if not impossible, to be in love with it. In not revering the spirit behind the plant, appreciating all its inexplicably beautiful powers, we lose out on the full benefit of the leaf, fruit, and root. The source of the plant's power is the same source for our healing and wellness, and we appear to be losing sight of both in our age of rampant technophilia.

Conscious eating—being fully present with food and the sensation of taste—is a crucial concept in many Eastern spiritual disciplines yet a novel concept to many Westerners. In American culture we are usually doing two or three other things while eating. I remember years ago eating in a lunch room sitting across from a Chinese woman who had lived in 17 countries on account of her husband's career. As she looked around the table at all of us doing some combination of eating, reading, watching TV, debating, and talking on a phone, she commented, "Americans are the only people I have ever seen who do so many other things than eat while they are eating." Yes, we love our multi-tasking capabilities, even if it means we go unaware of what we eat or how much of it really satisfies us.

Perhaps we really are missing the boat in this regard. Our American palate seems to be so desensitized to the subtleties of taste that intensely sweet and glaringly salty are the only two notes that our gustatory symphony can play and register as good. This taste-blindness, as I call it, severely limits our nutritional choices and our natural enjoyment of health-providing foods. We limit our vocabulary by learning only a few letters in the alphabet and then become perplexed by our health illiteracy.

If I received a two-dollar bill for every time someone asked me what vitamin or supplement they should take to be healthy, as though it were like taking some magic pill, my net worth might rival that of Bill Gates. People don't ask what foods they should be eating to fit them or how they could be preparing their meals to get optimal nutrition; neither do they inquire about exercise practices or ways to incorporate better breathing into their daily routines to better oxygenate their blood and brain. How about asking "Can I grow my own produce even if I am an apartment dweller?" There are ways to do it, yes. If you want a great choice in fresh produce, grow your own.

We need to redirect our efforts away from the thrill-of-the-pill mentality and get back to the basics of what really works. Some in the critical mass may dissent: "But pills are so quick, easy, and convenient." Pills do have their place. Sometimes pharmaceutical interventions are lifesavers, and when you are facing an emergency, they can be brilliant. The wise advice is not to neglect the day-to-day basics only to wake up when it is danger-zone time. You can do better and create better health through common-sense recommendations. Why set yourself up for an emergency?

Did you know that the foundation of all vitamin research comes from research of vitamins *in foods*? How many people who take vitamin supplements think that vitamins give them energy? Guess what? Vitamins do *not* give you energy—nutrients (carbohydrates, proteins, fats) do, as well as water and breathing. I will amend that list: connectin~ Spirit also energizes you. Do the research yourself, and you v that nothing surpasses the efficacy of the Big Three: (1) a good quality diet that fits your specific needs, (2) regular sensible exercise, and (3) some means for consistently connecting to Spirit.

Making the Commitment

So where does a person start? First, a variety of foods is needed. Easy enough, right? Some people interpret this statement in the following way: "Good news! Now I get to buy salt-and-vinegar potato chips, as well as barbeque, mesquite with ruffles, ketchup flavored, and nachos with cheese. This is variety, eh?" This is how the ego works, always trying to hedge the system in our favor. What is meant by a variety of foods and good nutrition is this:

a) Eat locally grown produce, as much variety as you can find or grow yourself.

b) Don't become a victim of habit and just eat the same five convenience foods each week (sound familiar?); your body needs a variety of quality nutrients. Stretch your comfort zone and try out new foods. This also means getting familiar with a wider array of tastes. I am amazed—no, shocked—when I see the diet journals that the classes complete (the ones who complete them honestly). Some people eat the same foods as a weekly habit; often they are fast foods or biologically dead convenience foods. If you are going to be repetitive, at least repeat with foods that have a benefit for your body.

c) Try new ways of preparing familiar foods. Once you enjoy the taste of steamed veggies, you cannot go back to the old way of boiling them to death, as my Southern mother was so adept at doing. (Sorry, Ma. You know I love you, but you frequently killed the corn and green beans. I didn't know this until the first time I actually tasted vegetables in their steamed preparation. "Wow! They are so crunchy. Is this what they really taste like?")

d) Eat foods that fit your metabolic needs. This is really not a chore as much as a journey of exploration and education. Some people thrive on good quality protein and fat, and others need complex carbohydrates. Others need a balanced combination of the two. One of the most difficult changes for most people to make is their eating habits. Eating sensibly does not mean suffering. There are those fast-food addicts who insinuate that I must be some kind of culinary masochist, getting by on raw leaves and sprouts, and someone who expects you to do the same. Yes, Virginia, you can eat good foods in agreeable combinations and enjoy your meals.

e) Try creative food combining. After repeated practice, you will notice a significant difference in how you feel after a meal. Excellence in your dietary choices should make you feel somewhat energized and revitalized by a meal, not heavy and lethargic. This means sensible combinations of foods as well as the right nutrients for you.

Emotions also play a crucial role in health, facilitating hyperacidity in the body or creating stress reduction and homeostasis. Pathogens seem to love most hyper-acidic environments, and chronic stress is a prime culprit of acidosis. *How* you eat is just as important as *what* you eat. Perhaps you have a father who used to chastise you and your sister at the dinner table with "We will have none of that negative talk during dinner!" It turns out that dad was right; it is very harmful to the process of digestion to be hostile or anxious during eating. Slow down, take your time, and get your mind and body doing the same thing—*receiving* nutrition. Distressing conversations, either from a person, a TV, or a radio have no place during a meal. Your entire gastrointestinal tract will thank you for adhering to that "old-fashioned" common-sense principle.

The connection between the mind and the body is crucial in our exploration in understanding foods and health. To paraphrase what Edgar Cayce once said in a reading, "What you think plus what you eat make who you are." So not only are you the result of your food choices, but you are equally your thought choices, as well. What do you feed your mind daily? Just as poor nutrition eventually leads to poor physical health, destructive mental habits lead to mental afflictions of one or another variety. These too can be transformed by starting productive habits. It is never too late.

The central point is not to become fanatical about foods but rather to be able to take a healthy, balanced approach to everyday living. Remember that *health* and *wholeness* mean the same thing.

It is vital to maintain optimal health through a sensible diet when you are recovering from illness or surgery, or if your immune system has been weakened for any reason. Understanding this also makes you a valuable source of knowledge if you ever serve in the role of caregiver to someone ailing. In this context, food acts as medicine.

As the sages of old knew, "It is much better to prevent an illness than to try to cure one." Bolstering your immunity through a good diet, regular exercise, connection to Spirit, and through managing stress is one of the most valuable gifts you can give to yourself and one of the oldest bits of philosophical wisdom still applicable today, just as it was in the era of the Chinese Yellow Emperor in the middle of the third millennium B.C.E. But as it often goes, knowing is one thing, but doing it is quite another. We have disease to lose and wholeness to gain. It is not a matter of how long you will live but rather *how* you live long.

1

The Holistic Legacy of Edgar Cayce

WHAT IMPRESSES THE GENERAL PUBLIC ABOUT MR. CAYCE'S LEGACY is how a man uneducated in medical science, who did not attend school past the eighth grade, could give a psychic reading diagnosing someone's health problem, often to a degree of accuracy that physicians of the day could not exceed. For people who actually followed through completely in applying the health advice, the cure rate was well above the statistical average.

Add to the health readings the litany of other topics covered by Mr. Cayce's work in the over fourteen thousand documented readings he gave for more than five thousand people—covering some forty years—and the scope of his gift to the world expands exponentially. Sixty years after Mr. Cayce's passing to spirit and we are still barely grasping the full implications of how we, as spirits in a physical world, can access a higher wisdom and implement that knowledge as pragmatically as the Cayce Source prompted.

It was his own self-healing that started his mission as the father of modern holism, along with seeking to heal his own son Hugh Lynn and his wife Gertrude. It was his ability to obtain healing information for diverse human conditions in such an extraordinary manner that impresses many. It is human nature that many perceive his legacy in a way that overrides the notion that Mr. Cayce's most impressive feat was his commitment to service.

It is easy to forget the tremendous personal price Mr. Cayce paid from the very beginning, after discovering his gift, and too easy to dismiss the continual strife that he and his family endured because of his commitment to helping others in need and being the best servant. Even the price he paid physically, giving an excessive number of readings during his ailing health because there were people in need, was a kind of self-sacrifice emulative of the Master's way.

Mr. Cayce was not a saint, at least not in the conventional sense, and his readings are not infallible, but perfection is not of this earth. We could take any profound document, from the U.S. Constitution to the Ramayana, and any person from Jesus to Gandhi, and find flaws if we look with a cynical eye. But if we, in the ethos of Zen Buddhism, accept the "perfect imperfection" of all teachings and teachers, we can begin to truly appreciate the legacy of Mr. Cayce's work.

What is most amusing to study in retrospect is how the Cayce Source, as it is commonly called, repetitively rebuked Cayce for not heeding the Source's advice for himself: for not spiritualizing his consciousness enough. After all, we suffer from the same predicament. May our desire to serve each other and do God's will be as determined as Mr. Cayce's was. It was his earnest wish to be of service to humanity with no thought of personal aggrandizement that was his most impressive feat.

What exactly did Mr. Cayce do to access the information called the Source? And what was it he accessed? To address this, we can only put pieces of the puzzle together to create a kind of philosophical Rorschach.

There seemed to be two events happening at any given reading. First, Edgar Cayce the man would lapse into a type of simulated coma, leaving his physical body, directing his consciousness towards his higher self. Once outside of time and space, other spiritual assistants such as a "keeper of the [akashic] records" would guide his higher self. The Akashic Records are an ancient Vedic era idea suggesting that all thoughts and events here on this earth are recorded upon a very fine substance called akasha, and these records can be accessed by those who know how to focus their mind and direct their spirit. Mr. Cayce accessed this huge library of events for multiple topics found in the readings. We can call this the introspective aspect.

Second, the readings were influenced by who was in the room at the time of the reading, including the person for whom the reading was given, the stenographer, and any friends and supporters. As Mr. Cayce left his body to get information for the client, he would also access the collective consciousness created by all attendees. It was akin to linking multiple databases together to have a better chance of getting clearer information about any given topic. If someone had knowledge of an aspect of the information needed for the reading, this psychic pool would be contacted to facilitate the desired goal of the request. This could also, at times, affect the language that was used or the quality of the reading.

Many things had an influence upon the quality of the readings—Mr. Cayce's physical health (and foods he would take), the sincerity and motive of the person asking for a reading, and the surreptitious motives of people in attendance, to name a few. We can call this the transpective aspect.

Often there was an intertwining of these two views, the introspective and the transpective. The database that Mr. Cayce would read into seemed to get more accessible as time progressed; the more you do something, the more proficient you become. The quality of the readings also benefited from the focus and sincerity of the inquirer.

Most of the Cayce readings, over 9000, are centered on physical healings. After all, if you are seriously ill, getting better is your number one priority; who you were in 1569 can wait until the bleeding stops.

The three main areas that comprise our self—body, mind, and spirit—are addressed consistently as being a unity (not a trinity) in the Source's physical healings. You need the soul to heal the body, to paraphrase the father of Western medicine, Hippocrates of Cos, and this is apparent when understanding the subject of healing.

Concerning the readings for the body, there are four subcategories that the Cayce Source consistently returns to: assimilation, circulation, elimination, and relaxation. These can be corroborated to a high degree by traditional Chinese medicine and Indian ayurveda.

Assimilation includes the type of nutrients taken, the combinations in which they are taken, and how the body digests the various properties. The mind was consistently mentioned as being needed for quality digestion. In other words, you cannot have your mind refracted upon five different tasks or ideas while you are eating and expect to get the most from your food, especially if focused upon the negative. This is contrary to the contemporary notion that multitasking is the best way to get work accomplished and that eating when upset may actually make you feel better.

We can pause here for a minute to contemplate the teachings of the great Vietnamese Zen master Thich Nhat Hanh. His teachings prompt us all to cultivate mindfulness for ourselves so that, in classic Buddhist tradition, you are aware—aware of what you are doing, why you are doing it, and to whom you are doing it. The majority of busy urban people are vague on all three points and probably do not consider the act of eating to be part of a spiritual practice. Thich Nhat Hanh teaches a simple and profound mindfulness exercise relating to eating[1]:

> "Contemplating your food—
> 'This plate of food,
> So fragrant and appetizing,
> Also contains much suffering.'"

Mindfulness here means awareness. Awareness means empathy with those around the globe who sacrifice themselves as laborers often under harsh conditions so that the luxuriant marketplaces of the industrialized West can offer African chocolate, South and Central American coffee, and Southeast Asian rice. When you pray for your food mindfully, you are praying for those people who labored with difficulty as well as all the people in the profit line, from farmer to exporter to grocery buyer. In Buddhist tradition, this is getting your heart and stomach right or, to employ an American vernacular, "gettin' all your cows headed on the same trail."

According to both the Cayce Source and ancient Eastern wisdom, you are less effective in any one thing when your attention is bifurcated or trifurcated, as it were. Your body needs your mental attention when you are taking nutrients, if you wish to get the most from your food.

Assimilation equals absorption of the food and of the vibration of the plant or animal.

Some Eastern teachers have noted that the widespread violence in the U.S. is energetically linked to (1) the violence that is in the meat supply that we abundantly consume (what we feed our bodies) and (2) the violence that we feed our minds with video games, television, and movies. One somewhat alters the vibration of the meat (or whatever nutrient) by practicing this mindful awareness recommended by Thich Nhat Hanh and in so doing makes the act of consuming a type of prayer.

The Cayce Source approaches this same issue from a slightly different slant. The basic idea is that God is everything but becomes altered or distorted through the activities of mankind. All material things have their inception as an idea, just as all physical phenomena are ideas of the Creator. Humans take these ideas and filter them first through an individual perception and then through a given cultural perception. The actual thing is always at least twice removed from its original nature. To see something as it truly is, we have to transcend both our cultural and personality biases. Although not impossible, it is not an easy task.

> When matter comes into being, what has taken place? The Spirit ye worship as God has moved in space and time to make for that which gives its expression; perhaps, as wheat, as corn, as flesh, as whatever may be the movement in that ye call time and space.   281-24

The movement referred to in this reading is what I alluded to, regarding both types of bias—both occurring "in space and time."

Assimilation is akin to digestion, and we cannot digest that which we are unable to receive. We cannot receive that which we are unaware of and ungrateful for. The timeless myth told by our assimilation is this: "[The Lord] has given food and provisions to those who worship and revere Him."[2] and "Heavenly Father, receive this, make it holy. Let no impurity of greed defile it. The food comes from Thee; it is for Thy temple. Spiritualize it. Spirit to Spirit goes."[3]

Circulation is what happens after assimilation, when nutrients hit your blood stream. It also refers to the larger context of cardiovascular and lymphatic circulation. You may think of the lymph in your body as the "white blood" with special vessels that transport lymphatic fluid through lymph nodes, which are especially congregated in your armpits and groin area. It is one of the numerous ways your body cleans out your tissues and blood stream. The lymph system does not have a pump like the cardiovascular system does, so muscular movement is needed to move lymph through the body.

One of the ways recommended to manually accomplish this pumping is through therapeutic massage. Massage therapy was recommended in the Cayce readings for numerous purposes, often to enhance the circulation of blood and lymph, to coordinate glandular and nervous activities, to work medicinal solutions into the body, and to compliment osteopathic adjustments.

Increasing circulation is one of the many things for which a good, therapeutic massage session can be beneficial. This is especially significant for anyone who is sedentary due to age or illness. The truth is that you will move about as much lymph in approximately eight to ten minutes of regular exercise as you would in fifty minutes of massage. However, if you cannot be ambulatory, massage is a useful substitute.

Circulation is crucial to healing. If you want to facilitate healing in the body, create sufficient blood flow; to increase healing, enhance blood flow.

Understanding this on the esoteric level, circulation is how you are in the world after assimilation. In other words, what good are you for the tribe? Another way of thinking about this is that assimilation is nourishment and survival, while circulation is activity and service. The heart is the center, the master, of the circulatory system. The timeless myth told by our circulation is "What comes around goes around," and it is a powerful story.

Well-functioning elimination is one of the most crucial processes necessary for good health. The Cayce readings refer to poor elimination as the cause of disease in many of the physical readings. This problem has been exacerbated since the early part of the twentieth century due to our increase of food additives, sedentary occupations, television culture, refined starches, and abundant processed food on our plates.

A fundamental way that your body removes dead cells is through bowel eliminations. Waste products accumulate faster in a system that is not having a daily bowel movement. This toxic backup, especially if chronic, is central to the start of numerous health problems. Here are four easy-to-do tasks that you can implement to naturally kick-start your body's valuable elimination functioning:

1. Eat more roughage, now called fibrous foods, twice a day. These include leafy greens, figs, dates, prunes, plant stalks and roots, flax seed meal, and oat or wheat bran. Even just taking raw fruit twice a day is a good start.

2. Drink more water! Somewhere between two and three liters a day. The more fiber you add to your diet, the more water you need to drink.

3. Massage your own abdomen, moving in a clockwise direction pressing in with a circular motion. You should try and pull in your abdominal muscles at the same time. You can also find a massage therapist who is trained in abdominal massage. Once you know what it feels like, you can perform the same maneuvers on your own body. It is safe and natural, and it works.

4. One of the oldest natural laxative tonics is hot water and freshly squeezed lemon first thing in the morning. This can be enhanced with fresh basil or cinnamon bark for an additional medicinal kick.

The other eliminative organs crucial to good health are your lungs. It is important to breathe deeply throughout the day, especially exhaling. All the Asian health arts from Taoist Kung Fu to yogic Pranayama focus intently on breathing. Ancient Chinese tradition speaks of the "elders who had long life because they breathed deeper than we do." This was written some twenty-three centuries ago, so we really have a lot of catching up to do. In Genesis 2:7, God "breathes into his [Adam's] nostrils the breath of life." Everything depends on breath. In many languages, breath and spirit mean the same thing or share the same word or character.

This is emblematic for the fact that we rely on the unseen for everything—body, mind, and soul. The timeless myth of our elimination is
"Let go and let God" and "In this world and the next / There is impurity
and impurity: / When a woman lacks dignity / When a man lacks gen-
erosity / But the greatest impurity is ignorance / Free yourself from it /
Be pure."[4]

The fourth subcategory of physical health to attend to diligently is
relaxation. Our modern vernacular would express this as stress management. Knowing how to eliminate the unnecessary stressors and
manage the ones that you cannot change is a necessary habit for good
health in our frenetic, ever-kinetic Information Age.

The Cayce Source returned to emotions repeatedly as potential
sources of disease. This knowledge is also an integral part of understanding health and healing in traditional Chinese medicine and Indian
ayurveda. Our modern technophilic system is the first medical model
that separates the functioning of the body from the mind. With the
increasing study in a relatively new medical discipline that explores the
relationships between the mind and the immune system, psychoneuro-
immunology, the post-industrial medical behemoth is coming back to
ancient traditions. Welcome back aboard. The rather regrettable effect
of this happening within the confines of a chemocentric medical culture is that pills will likely be the resulting solution to the problem of
the month. Let us hope this will change with the entrance into medical
school of more holistically oriented healers and future medical pio-
neers. I am hopeful it will.

We know chronic stress is a killer, whether it is physical or mental.
The Buddha has famously stated that your mind is the most important
aspect of your personality to develop, since your world is filtered
through the quality of your consciousness. Here are some words of
wisdom from a being who figured this out:[5]

1. "Your worst enemy cannot harm you as much as your own
thoughts, unguarded. But once mastered, no one can help you as
much, not even your father or your mother."

2. "Are you quiet? Quiet your body. Quiet your mind. You want
nothing. Your words are still. You are still. By your own efforts

waken yourself, watch yourself, and live joyfully."
3. "To straighten the crooked you must first do a harder thing—
    straighten yourself."

What can you do about managing stress? Ask yourself, "In a hundred
years, will this really matter?" The Cayce Source enjoyed the phrase,
"Watch oneself go by." This is another way of getting perspective, of
stepping outside of your little drama and seeing that you are not really
the earth's axis. The world goes on, with or without you. While you are
here, do your best, not someone else's worst; be kind and patient; sur-
render to Spirit. Learn to meditate—the best means to get to know the
real you, the one behind all the "sturm and drang" of this world created
by the mind.

The timeless myth of our relaxation is "Be still and know that I am
God."[6]

The legacy of the Cayce Source is manifold. For the purpose of understanding health and healing, it is valuable to keep in mind the basics:

•   Good foods are needed for good health.

•   Watch what you feed your mind even more than what you feed
your stomach, but have a sensible diet.

•   Pay attention to the big four: assimilation, circulation, elimination, and relaxation.

•   You cannot genuinely heal the body without engaging the soul,
so engage the soul daily.

•   Be of good use in this world—serve your fellow humans. The difference you make, no matter how small, is great in the eyes of God.

•   In giving, you get; in surrendering, you are supported; in loving,
you are loved. To paraphrase the Dalai Lama, "You should help each
other, but if you cannot help each other, do not hurt each other."

2

The Fleshy Machine

IT IS QUITE ASTOUNDING TO DISCOVER THE LARGE NUMBER OF
people who do not know their body–not to the degree of a medical
specialist or health professional but just the basics–the ability to confi-
dently answer the question "Where are the spleen, stomach, liver, and
colon located?" If the plumbing, electricity, air conditioning, or heating
unit in your house malfunctions, you should know where the equip-
ment is in order to repair it, and I suspect that most people know more
about their house than their own fleshy machine.

The most important factor in understanding how the body stays in
balance (or does not) is the nervous system, specifically the autonomic
nervous system and the cerebrospinal nervous system. These are not
really separate systems, as no organ or tissue system functions completely independently; they are two sides of the same coin. When your
body is in balance, in a state of ease, technically called homeostasis (or
conversely, when out of balance and in a state of dis–ease), these two
systems are functioning harmoniously.

The nervous system is the electrical medium between thoughts, ideas,
and perceptions, all occurring in the mind, and the physical housing,
principally the myofascial–skeletal system. The nervous system is the
vehicle for translating thought into action and spirit into soma.[1]

The health of the nervous system is predicated upon good nutrition,
which includes nutrients rich in quality fat–soluble and water–soluble
vitamins. Your diet, coupled with how well you manage stressors (your

mental diet), helps predict the state of your nervous system. Your nervous system is the center of all other biological functions, affecting all organs, as well as the endocrine (glandular), digestive, and myofascial-skeletal systems.

The nervous system is separated into two main divisions, the cerebrospinal system and the autonomic system, which play off each other in day–to–day activities and perceptions.

The cerebrospinal division includes the brain and spinal cord, and all the nerves that attach to your limbs. This division is responsible for voluntary functioning of the body. The principle job of the cerebrospinal division is moving the fleshy machine here and there with force, grace, urgency, style, rhythm—all the ways that one uniquely expresses himself or herself through movement and posture. This is how a person willfully moves through space.

The autonomic (another term for *automatic*) division includes nerve ganglia (networks) that lie parallel to the spine on both sides. This division is responsible for the mostly involuntary processes of the body, such as respiration, myocardial functioning and circulation, and peristalsis,[2] to identify just a few. The standard medical orthodoxy considers this division to be wholly involuntary and not significantly influenced by the will, but by emotional reactions only.

The ancient Asian traditions that produce advanced yogis, swamis, and lamas present a counterpoint to this modern orthodox idea. Many of these Asian adepts have been documented slowing their heartbeat to a standstill and slowing down respiration to such a degree that they can be buried for days and weeks underground only to be exhumed and found to be biologically fully functional. The great swami Paramahansa Yogananda writes about just a few of these adepts in his classic book *Autobiography of a Yogi*.[3] There are numerous examples available for one to study.

The medical clairvoyant Edgar Cayce, along with the father of osteopathic medicine, A.T. Still, and respected Eastern teachers from B.K.S. Iyengar to Baba Hari Dass all concur on the importance of coordinating these two divisions of the nervous system: the voluntary and involuntary. It is the chronic discord between these two that facilitates many diseases.

What are some ways to remedy or, better yet, prevent this discord? A fantastic starting point would be to learn meditation and practice regularly. This is an outstanding method for gaining mind–body, cerebrospinal–autonomic harmony. Secondly, moderate your stress levels and cultivate methods to effectively handle stressors: allow more time for travel and commuting, do not take it all so seriously, and learn how to stop the "monkey mind" from perpetuating its crazy little agenda. Thirdly, get your eating habits on track. Eating good quality fats, produce raised in nutritious soil, and foods naturally high in C and B–complex vitamins, knowing your metabolic dominance (carbohydrate–, protein–, or mixed–type dominance), minimizing (or better yet, eliminating) refined sugars and starches, and drinking plenty of purified water will greatly enhance your health and well–being.

Even though the body is exceedingly resilient under most circumstances, there is a point of no return if you abuse yourself long enough. There are certain conditions of disease in which the catabolic or tearing–down functions of the cellular matrices are dominating the anabolic or building–up functions of the cells. If the underlying imbalance is not discovered early enough and treated properly, the above recommendations may be palliative at best.

The role stress plays in the perpetuation of disease cannot be overstated. A person who is always stressed out or a chronic nervous wreck will surely manifest an illness, as the autonomic and cerebrospinal systems cannot function well in disharmony. This is simply your body's way of getting your attention to make a change. All the various symptoms of disease are gifts from the marvelous intelligence of your body alerting you that you are somehow out of balance. How you remedy the situation is up to your free will and common sense.

Every credible educator and researcher acknowledges this next point, even if there is not accord on any other detail: regular exercise is medicine for your body and mind and is excellent for naturally reducing stress levels while increasing your body's stress adaptation ability.

What is good exercise? Here we may have diverging opinions, but undoubtedly one can rely on this definition: *Moving the body with awareness and enthusiasm*. A daily brisk walk does many good things for the body. Do not push it too far with exercise—just enough so that there is perspiration and a slight feeling of exhilaration. We are made to move the body with awareness and enthusiasm, whatever our age.

The sedentary life is a real killer. We are tied to our desks and computers five out of seven days during the sun's best hours—forty, fifty, sixty hours a week. Certainly our evolutionary trajectory is thrown off a bit by this, being that we have worked much harder to accumulate our food supplies in the not-too-distant past. Add to this sedentary dilemma poor nutrition, which is becoming more common all the time with people's frantic, overscheduled lives, with fewer people growing their own produce or raising their own animals for food. It seems we are verging on an epidemic of lethargy and dietary malaise, all the while over-relying on technology to show us the way.

Our post-industrial culture has created the habit of eating convenient empty-calorie foods on the run, with no thought of the essence or quality of the nutrient, with substitutes galore: fat substitutes, sugar substitutes, taste substitutes. After all, who really wants to eat cardboard sprinkled with paprika, conveniently available in a nearby vending machine, if it is not going to be chemically enhanced? If we add to this equation more refined sugar consumption per person than we have seen in the last two-hundred-plus years of sugar's ignoble appearance in commercial food and drink supplies, we are set up for a Casey Jones nervous system train wreck.

Take care of the body's nervous system: everything depends on its healthy functioning—organs, muscles, glands, hormones, and especially your spirit.

The next intriguing system to explore briefly is the myofascial–skeletal system. The body's myofascia is the combination of the intricate connective tissue network (fascia) and muscle tissue (the Latin root for which is *myo* or *mya*). Covering every bone, organ, vein, artery, vessel, tendon, ligament, and muscle is the pervasive and sturdy tissue called fascia.[4] Understanding fascia is crucial to understanding the integrity and long-term health of your entire biologic network.

Since fascia envelops all structures of the body, it interacts significantly with all structures. We cannot get a reliable sense of this by examining fascia on cadavers but only in vivo. By the time the body expires, fascia has already started dehydrating, and the crucial life energy that flows through fascia quickly dissipates.

Fascia is a dynamic, living system that can only be truly appreciated in living bodies. You may think of it as the Saran Wrap of all the tissues of the body—it is covering everything from your skull to your palms to your soles, deep to superficial. It is made up of three substances that rely considerably on nutritional sources for repletion and regeneration: collagen, hyaline, and ground substance. Collagen is a protein that has many uses in the body. It is widely known as an injectable substance used by models and entertainers to puff up their lip size (as in "I just had my lips done, dahling"). Yes, they are getting injections of animal collagen. Where else has a person encountered collagen? In commercial gelatin (about 40–45% collagen) and upon the ends of chicken bones; that opaque gristle-like material is made of collagen.

Currently there are about twenty-one types of collagen used in medical or cosmetic applications, in everything from catheters, corneal implants, and artificial skin (for skin grafts) to the cosmetic kind with which Paulina Pouter gets her lip tissue distended. And yes, most of it comes from animal tissue. I wonder if the vegan supermodel knows that? The next time you see the model with the ballooned high-fashion lips, just think—her lip stuffing could have been the posterior loin of a common Hereford. Ah, the price to pay for beauty.

Not only do the soft tissues of the body have a fascial wrapping (muscles, tendons, and the like), but all the bones of the body do, too. The skeletal system acts as the dynamic support, the moving framework, for the myofascial system. It is also an important production center for red and white blood cells in the bone's marrow and the most abundant storage system for calcium and phosphorus. Almost two-thirds of the weight of a bone is calcium phosphate, the two most plentiful minerals in the body. The majority of remaining third is collagen, and collagen components, the building block of connective tissue (fascia).

All life implies movement. This system of your muscles, connective tissues, and skeleton, which is referred to here as the myofascial-skeletal system, is the prime source of movement, of life. One of the essential functions of nutrition is to provide energy for the neuromuscular system (nervous + muscular tissues) and quality tissue production for the myofascial–skeletal system. If your nutritional habits are sub–par, your body will eventually reveal this in the myofascial–skeletal system in many possible manifestations of disease: osteoporosis, osteomalacia, fibromyalgia, persistent muscle cramps, postural deviations, gout, osteoarthritis. And the list has just begun.

One of the misleading aspects of studying the body as separate organ systems, organs, and tissues is that this approach can easily convey the illusion of biologic independence. The truth is that the body operates as a whole unit, and it always has. Each organ system—nervous, muscular, skeletal, fascial—is a separate "finger" connecting to one "hand." It is important to emphasize this as one studies individual functioning and specific relationships of systems. A greater understanding of the various organ systems of the body inevitably leads the individual back to the concept of oneness: everything depends upon everything else.

The body is so complex in each individual system that modern medicine has developed specific disciplines to keep track of each area. A person sees a specialist for heart conditions, another for brain and nervous conditions, another for glandular disease, and yet another to work with the mind. Some contend that in this expanding field of separate medical specialties, the right medical hand may not know what the left medical hand is doing.

This is significant and comes to the public's attention when, for example, one physician prescribes medication for a person's ailment and another specialist, without the knowledge of the first physician's prescription, recommends the patient take another pill for a different (although perhaps related) ailment. The interaction of these two chemicals, known as an iatrogenic reaction, causes difficulties and even considerable fatalities in some cases.[5] There is no way for the chemical companies that produce these drugs to account for all the possible biochemical interactions, although software has recently been developed for pharmacists to warn them if a patient is taking multiple medications with possible dangerous interactive effects. Confucius says: The wise one does not completely put his fate in the hands of a computer program.[6]

The last area of investigation in understanding the fleshy machine is the digestive system, which starts with the three pairs of salivary glands in the mouth and terminates at the rectum, the final aspect of the large intestine.

When one eats carbohydrates, especially starches, there is a substantial amount of saliva required to properly digest that nutrient. What is very common with many people is washing down starches with liquids after a few chews. This is a highly inefficient way to digest starches. Starches require enzymes produced in the parotid glands to start turning the polysaccharide (multi-chained sugar, another name for a starch) into smaller saccharides, tri-, di-, and eventually monosaccharides (single unit sugars, also called simple sugars). The digestive system does this with all nutrients—transforms them from their complex form to their simplest form. Proteins become amino acids, and fats become fatty acids in the same manner. The foremost difference between the three major nutrients is that starches need lots of saliva for efficient digestion, especially if you are a person who already gets an upset stomach easily or excess stomach acidity, heartburn, etc. If this is you, then chew, chew, and chew.

For the average person, drinking small sips of liquid during a meal should not pose a problem; just be aware of not washing down food with liquids. The old-fashioned advice on this subject is still valid, although it should not be thought of as a gospel rule: drink liquids 20-30 minutes prior to a meal and 20 minutes after a meal. A variety of people who have applied this rule have reported very favorable results.

Besides the glands in the mouth breaking down starches, there are glands in the stomach that secrete acids to break down proteins and some fats. You would likely discover that if you ate one nutrient at a time this would facilitate optimal digestion—eating meat without anything else, for example—but this is unrealistic for most people. What is reasonable for most is to be aware of what nutrient is dominant in any given meal. Knowing your metabolic dominance plays a significant part in paying attention to what nutrient you are having the most of. If you are a protein-dominant type, you want to minimize (although not necessarily eliminate) your starches and, equally advisable, not eat sugars at the same time as meats. If you are a carbohydrate-dominant type, you want to maximize the fat-starch combinations and keep the protein portions smaller.

For a healthy person, especially for most under thirty-five, many nutrients in small portions can be combined at a meal without noticeable ill effects. For people who may have health concerns or who are enduring disease, being mindful of food combinations would be a very prudent course to take. (Refer to chapters 7 and 8.)

Your stomach is an expansive receptacle that mixes acids and other complex chemicals with your food. It works to break down organic constituents into a stomach smoothie, called chyme, which your small intestine can receive. You have seen this stomach smoothie before: with yourself, the last time you had the stomach flu, and with your neighbor, weak-stomached Willy, the last time you got on the Tilt-A-Whirl at the carnival with him.

When the food you eat gets chemically reduced into chyme, a signal is sent through the autonomic nervous system to move food along and open the pyloric sphincter at the end of your stomach. This is a smooth muscle "door" that allows approximately 1 to 1.5 teaspoons of food at a time to pass into your small intestine.

In the small intestine most of the assimilation occurs. This is where food becomes energy or building material. If the body does not require energy or building material, it will (a) get rid of it or (b) store it. Since the body is so intelligent, ("Get ready, here comes another plate full!") it will likely opt for the latter. It assumes that a person is eating six meals a day for a reason: perhaps pregnancy or storing up for a long, hard winter. If a person is overweight because of careless portion control, the body cannot be in blame but just may be, in time, embalmed. Confucius says: "Don't let the spoon dig your own grave."

After the crucial functioning of the small intestine, which in some people can reach thirty to thirty-three feet in length (or more), food then passes to the large intestine, also known as the colon. This is where the final water-absorption phase occurs as well as bacterial digestion of any leftover nutrients.

The fleshy machine is a complex one. Since there are so many areas to consider when separating the whole into components, there are three primary areas that one can focus on to jump-start health: the nervous system, the myofascial-skeletal system, and the digestive system. Coordinating the active and restful branches of the nervous system is central to many health traditions around the world. Let us not be so haughty to think that because a system is ancient or uses a different biological or psychosomatic map than our present post-industrial one that it is inferior. Western medicine shares the same holistic roots as the Asian systems through the ancient Greeks. There are millions of people at present enjoying good health by following these ancient traditions and millions who have thrived in the past. In understanding the fleshy machine we benefit from everyone's outlook, old and new. Let each person decide for himself or herself what the best course to take might be, but let us not limit our choices based on an ill-informed prejudice or bureaucratic myopia.

Although not the only way, one of the best habits for coordinating the nervous system is through regular meditation. This simple (but often challenging) discipline, coupled with stress management and a good quality diet, is paramount to good health. It is also important to have a basic understanding of how your body functions. The more you learn, the more informed you are to make worthwhile choices. The next step, as the Eastern traditions teach, is to get to the root of the mind, the source of the body's purpose.

3

Physiology Fundamentals

MANY PEOPLE CAN EXPLAIN HOW A COMPUTER, AUTOMOBILE, OR airplane operates, but when asked about their own body, their most precious vehicle, they often are clueless. How strange that we should invest so much effort in knowing machines and so little in knowing our own bodies. The following paragraphs should establish the basics.

Digestion and assimilation of nutrients is a complex process, and the various organ functions that support these processes also have many aspects to them. The following explanation is pared down for the sake of expediency, yet it is still a good starting point for understanding what is happening both when you eat and while you live.

The Mouth

You have three sets of salivary glands in the mouth that perform two important functions: (1) Secreting saliva that acts as both a lubricant for food and as a trap for bacteria. It is the chewing of food, mixing ample saliva with the nutrients, that helps isolate minor pathogens. This assumes, of course, that your immune system has not been deeply compromised. (2) Secreting a special enzyme called *alpha amylase (ptyalin)* that breaks down starches.

This is the first place in the body where starches get broken down, so it is important to chew starchy foods well to ease the burden on the rest of the digestive system. Starches, also called complex carbohydrates, need to be turned into sugars initially in the mouth. It is common for people to wash down breads and pastas with liquids, not allowing for this vital sugar breakdown, and this could have counterproductive consequences later in the digestion process. Breads are chewy for a reason; they need lots of saliva and chewing activity to prepare them for the small intestine, efficiently releasing the long–chain sugars.[1] Don't wash down starches or any nutrients with liquids.

As a result of numerous inquiries in class such as "How many times are we supposed to chew starches before we swallow them?" and replying that there is no number set by the International Board of Mastication, we can assume that grandma's advice to "chew thirty times before swallowing" is more than sufficient.

The Stomach

Nutrients do not get assimilated in the stomach. The stomach is a type of holding tank for food, preparing it for the small intestine, where about 90% of the nutritive assimilation occurs. The stomach's job is to create various acids and other chemicals to turn food into a kind of stomach smoothie called chyme (starts with "k" and rhymes with *lime*). There is a churning in the stomach caused by small muscular contractions (similar to the way a concrete truck mixes cement), rolling food over and mixing it with stomach acids. The stomach has folds in it that expand, somewhat like an accordion, to allow more room for that third helping of lasagna. If one overdoes it, a signal eventually gets sent from the lower part of the stomach saying, "No mas, no mas" [no more, no more], and that "accordion" plays a very mournful version of Lady of Spain, which your body interprets as digestive unhappiness.

There is a bit of a delay from the time when the brain registers being full from the special receptors in the stomach—all the more reason to eat slowly and observe the Three–Quarters Rule: Eat three–fourths as much as you think you want, stopping three–fourths before you want to. This is another reason for not getting too distracted during a meal, so you can pay attention to your body's signals and stop before it is too late.

The Small Intestine

The stomach terminates into this crucial organ. Here is Digestion Central. The average small intestine is about 20 feet long.[2] It has lots of little folds that have little finger–like projections on them, which in turn have smaller hair–like projections on them. All of this is for the purpose of creating more surface area in your body for nutrients to get broken down into energy or structure (muscle, fat, and so forth). If your small intestine were just a simple hollow tunnel, it would have a total absorptive surface of about 3.6 ft.[2] Instead, because of all the folds and projections atop projections, it has a total absorptive surface area of about 2200 ft![2] Baseball players tell me that is approximately the size of a standard baseball infield.

The small intestine occupies most of your abdominal region. A plethora of digestive enzymes and juices created by the liver and pancreas are mixed here with chyme, which then get absorbed into your bloodstream.

The Large Intestine

Also known as the colon, the large intestine has no enzymes released in it. Any digestion that occurs here is the result of both small intestine enzymes continuing to work and the activity of bacteria. An important function of the colon is the reabsorption of water and some of the B vitamins. If the colon does not reabsorb water, the result is diarrhea.

This is where the very important fecal material is formed. A bowel movement is composed of approximately 75% water, 5% bacteria, with the remaining 20% fiber, dead cells, and cellular waste products.

When starches go partially digested, because of poor food combining or excess fiber consumption, for example, there is a stimulation of excess bacterial gas (a.k.a. flatulence), which could facilitate cramping and abdominal distention. As a result of poorly digested sugars becoming food for the colon's bacteria, a very undesirable condition in the colon could manifest with symptoms as diverse as chronic fatigue, headaches, blurry vision, and skin problems.

You've Gotta Move

Having a healthy daily elimination is crucial to good health. No matter what supplements you take, how much you exercise, how long you watch your favorite yoga tapes, if you are not having a daily elimination, you are not healthy. Twice a day is even more efficient. A healthy BM should be well formed and in one piece, not in "marbles" or small fragments. There should not be any intense, offensive odor, as that may indicate a toxic environment of the colon's rectal columns. It is important to achieve the proper balance of healthy intestinal bacteria. Any chronic imbalances in this area could lead to other problems, the least of which is a very malodorous elimination. Of course, it is not going to smell like gardenias, but it should not make the hallway smoke detector activate either. You get the picture.

The Liver

Your liver is located on the right side of your body, behind your rib cage. This is the largest visceral organ in the body, weighing an average of 3–3.5 lbs. Some textbooks and clinical manuals attribute over two hundred functions to the liver. It is an extremely important organ, being the prime blood cleanser in the body. All toxins get filtered out in the liver, even medications, which the liver often sees as a foreign substance and tries to eradicate. This is why you have to keep taking a medication every 2 or 4 hours: your liver is getting rid of it for you.

Here is a short list of the many things your amazing liver does daily:

- Stores iron, just in case you need some extra that the blood does not have an abundance of. This is why eating the liver of animals is considered a rich dietary source of iron. Be very cautious—remember that the liver is filtering out toxins in the blood and all toxic materials that an animal ingests will also be stored in the liver. If you are going to eat organ meats, be very selective and know your source. If in doubt, leave it out.
- Stores fat–soluble vitamins A, D, E, and K. When your body needs extra, the liver has the supply. Recall that anything in excess the body likes to store.

- Helps regulate cholesterol levels and other blood fats.
- Stabilizes blood sugar levels. Working with the pancreas, blood sugar (glucose, via the hormone glucagon) and insulin levels are regulated by the liver.
- Manufactures bile (approximately one liter daily), which your body needs to break down fats. The liver's little neighbor to the south, the gall bladder, will store and concentrate the bile, which will be released as needed in the small intestine. You can still function without a gall bladder, but you will have to alter your intake of dietary fats and support your endocrine system with the right nutrients. Good dietary choices, food combining, and anti-oxidant support are key in this case.

The Pancreas

On the left side of your body, behind your stomach, lies your pancreas. It is an elongated, cigar–shaped organ approximately six inches in length with a nodular surface. This organ has two major jobs: (1) To produce a very alkaline substance called pancreatic juice, which is very rich in digestive enzymes. These enzymes break down fats, proteins, and starches. The amylase, the starch–specific enzyme, is almost identical to the amylase found in the saliva. In effect, when your mouth starts watering, so does your pancreas. (2) To secrete insulin, a hormone that keeps blood sugar levels regulated, and glucagon, a hormone that keeps blood sugar levels from being too deficient. It is a kind of yin–yang of the body (one of many)—when one goes down, the other rises, and vice–versa. Diabetics who take insulin shots cannot produce their own insulin in the pancreas, and their blood sugar levels can easily become excessive. When you eat a lot of refined sugar, your pancreas produces significant amounts of insulin to keep you in balance. At some point, the pancreas can "burn out" and lose its natural insulin or glucagon functioning. Some scientists think this is what may be happening in certain cases of adult–onset diabetes, where there is a strong dietary influence.

There is a lot more to the body, of course, but this is just a basic survey of the significant organs involved in digestion. It is good to be mindful of all the processes involved in turning food into your health—all the more reason to choose quality nutrients, take your time, chew well, think positive thoughts, and observe the Three–Quarters Rule.

4

Three Main Nutrients

THE MAJORITY OF FOODS WE EAT ARE A MIXTURE OF THE THREE PRI-
mary macronutrients: protein, fat, and carbohydrates. Steak, for example, is thought of as being a pure protein. The main ingredient in a
steak, however, is water, at about 59%, followed by protein, about 32%,
then fat at about 8%, all depending upon the type and cut of the meat.
Water, although a macronutrient, gets its own special category as a
unique nutritional substance. When a food is designated as fat or protein, this refers to what nutrient is most dominant. Cheese is dominant
in fat but does have some protein in it and a slight amount of carbohydrate. We therefore consider cheese a fatty food.

The following will briefly explain the major nutrients and some
sources for each.

Protein

Derived from the Greek root for *first, protos,* (as in *prototype* and *proto-
plasm*) *protein* refers to the most essential nutrient for building structure,
facilitating growth, and repairing tissues. As a matter of fact, your body
is basically one giant protein matrix, being that protein is the bulk of
muscle tissue, blood, connective tissues (for example, fascia, tendon,
ligament), hormones, antibodies, and enzymes.

All proteins are composed of carbon, hydrogen, oxygen, and nitrogen. It is the inclusion of nitrogen that distinguishes proteins from fat

and carbohydrates. The smallest functional unit in protein is an amino acid. There are about twenty common amino acids in total, but only nine are considered essential and are given the plausible title, *essential amino acids*. The body requires a dietary source for these nine essential amino acids. A chain of amino acids creates a distinctive protein structure called a peptide, or when many peptides glue together, a polypeptide.

Since meats can create either an acidic or alkaline reaction according to metabolic type, it is recommended that you know your metabolic requirements relative to protein intake. There is more value for the use of animal proteins when you are recovering from a major surgery or injury, when you need to repair and rebuild tissue. This is why chicken soup, a.k.a. "Jewish penicillin," has been popular for recovering from colds, illness, and physical trauma. The large amount of calcium–phosphorus coupled with the amino acids in the muscle tissue is ideal for somatic recovery and reparation, especially for protein–dominant metabolic types. You can recover with vegetable protein, however: a soup made from carrots, leeks, garlic, parsley, cilantro, millet and almond butter is a nice recovery broth, one that carbohydrate–dominant metabolic types especially appreciate. There is also the old standby of miso soup to rely upon, made of fermented soybean paste.

Protein Sources:
Animal–based
- Eggs
- Milk (including cheese, yogurt, and other)
- Muscle tissue (usually just known as meat, but yes, you are eating the muscles and connective tissues of an animal when you eat steak, chicken legs, and pork loin)
- Blood (Numerous cultures eat the blood of animals, raw and cooked.)
- Organ (visceral) meats: spleen, liver, heart, brain, glands, and other
- Gristle (often the cartilage, ligament, tendon, and the like; all the collagen–rich connective tissues of the animal)

Vegetable–based
- Legumes: soybeans, split peas, lima beans, dried beans, peanuts, nut butters

- Grains: corn, steel cut oats, wheat, brown rice, millet, quinoa, amaranth, buckwheat, and wild rice

It used to be thought that legumes and grains were not complete proteins in themselves—that is, they did not contain all the essential amino acids. Contemporary research indicates that whole grains do indeed comprise a complete protein. You get a very hearty, complete vegetable protein when you mix a legume with a whole grain. This combination is sometimes referred to as a light protein, distinguishing it from a heavy protein, a flesh- or visceral-based type, which requires many more stomach acids to digest. Light proteins are nutritious and much needed for carbohydrate-dominant types when they are trying to build muscle mass or to bolster their immune system (which should be ongoing maintenance).

This legume and whole grain combination is a dietary staple for many impoverished regions of the globe that cannot afford the luxury of growing animals for food. Eating a vegetable-based diet to fulfill your protein requirements is a logical choice for lowering your cholesterol levels and taking care of your circulatory system, especially if you are a slow oxidizer or a sympathetic-dominant metabolic type. The right lifestyle choices such as exercising, quitting smoking, and managing stress will also create a similar effect. Put the two together—light proteins and healthful lifestyle choices—and you have a well-known winner.

Proteins occur in nature often with fats, which is why a protein and fat food combination works well, especially for fast oxidizers and parasympathetic-dominant metabolic types.

Fats

Fats have received a bad reputation in the popular press. Some health educators have suggested that this is a purposeful ploy to hoodwink you into buying fat substitutes, thinking they are a more healthful choice. In most cases the faux-fat is worse for you than the real thing. It is recommended that you just eat the real thing, but in modest quantities.

What is so great about fats?

1. Fats carry the flavor of foods, and your body registers the message "I'm full" with digestion of these valuable nutrients. There are special receptors in the tongue, stomach, and small intestine that send signals to your brain that you are satiated. If you eat fat, you feel full faster with a smaller amount of ingested materials. Because of this, a little quality fat goes a long way. It is much easier to overeat when you are consuming foods made with fat substitutes or artificially engineered to be non-fat.[1] Your body does not register full as fast, and your spoon just keeps on scooping. Eat fat. It is good for you, and your body needs it. Consult the list of quality fats below for the best nutritional choices.

2. Fats are a very rich source of energy, more than double that of proteins and carbohydrates. They are absorbed more slowly than the other two nutrients, staying with you longer. If you have a short time to eat, like a short break at work, it is best to have some good quality fat; it will sustain you for a longer time than empty carbohydrates, and you will likely not eat as much when your next meal opportunity arises. Of course, you always have the free will to override your body's natural signals, which causes problems in the long term. If you are not very hungry, eat only a little. If you are not hungry at all, do not eat just to be social. If you have a short time to eat and need sustaining energy, include good fats.

3. Fats transport and store the fat-soluble vitamins A, D, E, and K. Taking these vitamins as a supplement without the presence of a quality food source of fats is essentially a waste of time and money, as your body will not utilize them well.

4. All your cells are made of fat. Together with protein, they constitute the structural framework of your body, from smallest to biggest. Certain fats assist with membrane suppleness, as well as help normalize nutrient transfer into and out of cells. They act as insulators, energy conduits, and nutrient reserves for your nervous and circulatory systems. In order for your nervous, endocrine, and cardiovascular systems to function optimally, your body re-

quires good quality fats; the emphasis here is *good quality*.

Types of fats

The primary building blocks of fats are fatty acids. The two essential fatty acids, linoleic acid and alpha-linoleic acid, are components of certain cell membranes and hormones.

Fats come in two major varieties: saturated and unsaturated. A saturated fat is one that has a surplus of hydrogen atoms clinging to carbon atoms within the fatty acid; the more hydrogen, the more saturated the fat is. These fats tend to be solid or semi-solid at room temperature (for example, cheese, butter, yogurt, palm oil, coconut oil). The fats that have less hydrogen atoms hanging on to their carbon neighbors are called unsaturated and are liquid at room temperature (vegetable oils).

Just when you thought we were done with the technicalities, there is more.

Unsaturated fats are classified by the relationships of carbon to hydrogen. If only one carbon-carbon bond is saturated with hydrogen, it is called monounsaturated. Olive and canola oils are examples of monounsaturated fats. If two or more carbon-carbon bonds are replete with hydrogen, this is known as a polyunsaturated fat. All the other vegetable oils besides olive and canola are polyunsaturated fats (for example, safflower, soybean, sesame).

A *really* unsaturated fat is fish oil, which is composed of omega-3 fatty acids, having six carbon-carbon bonds. (I know. We now have more bonds than an Ian Fleming film festival.) Fish that have their zip code in cold waters retain the highest amounts of omega-3 fatty acids; the six sites of saturation function as a type of antifreeze, keeping the mackerel from becoming a mackerel-sicle. Research has shown that eating cold-water fish, with its inherent omega-3 fats, can impart protection against stroke, heart attack, and heart disease. Many native North American tribes who have traditionally depended upon salmon consider it a sacred food because of the health-promoting quality of these fish fats and proteins.

This does not work the same with fish oil capsules, which have shown in some cases to be counterproductive, even dangerous. This is likely because it is easy to overdo capsules and take them without the ancillary nutrients to properly process the intensely rich oils.

The double-edged sword here is that even though cold-water fish is healthy for you, it has become challenging to locate fish supplies not contaminated with mercury and other reckless by-products of seaside or seafaring industries.[2]

Good Sources of Fat:
- Cold-water fish (mackerel, herring, Atlantic and sockeye salmon, tuna, sturgeon, and other)
- Olive oil and canola oil
- Organic butter (yes, it is superior to margarine)
- Cheese (soft and hard varieties, including cottage cheese and cream cheese)
- Free-range organic eggs (more fat in the white, more protein in the yolk)
- Nuts and nut butters (almond butter is one of the best choices)
- Meats (the more unprocessed and affected by commercial additives, the better)

When Fats Turn Ugly

Hydrogenation is a chemical process in which unsaturated fats are transformed into saturated fats by injecting the former with copious amounts of hydrogen. You have read the ingredients of the commercial cupcakes you love to secretly indulge in and found "partially hydrogenated vegetable oil" often among the top five ingredients. This hydrogenation process increases the shelf life of the product. Real butter will go rancid in time (without refrigeration), and chemically hydrogen-impregnated vegetable oil alleviates this problem and, according to the food industry, will taste just as delectable months, perhaps years, from the day it was created. Margarines and shortenings are produced through this hydrogenation process as a low-cost preservation method for baked goods.

The ensuing problem is that the unsaturated fatty acid gets mutated in the process of hydrogenation. The naturally occurring form of the fatty acid, called a *cis* form, basically a spiraling molecular structure, gets involuntarily straightened out. The mutant post–hydrogenation form, the straight version, is called a *trans fatty acid* and is well–documented as causing higher LDL cholesterol levels and elevating risks for heart disease. So stick with organic butter and shun the margarines— butter is better; just keep to slender portions.

Carbohydrates

Carbohydrates come from plants. There are three primary groups of carbohydrates, casually known as *carbs*. As we will discover, not all carbs are equal.

- Group One: Simple Sugars (a.k.a. saccharides)
- Group Two: Complex Carbohydrates (a.k.a. starches)
- Group Three: Dietary Fiber (a.k.a. roughage)

The Group One collection of carbs is the most immediately usable form for energy from foods. They break down to blood sugar (glucose) quite fast. The cast of simple sugars, glucose, fructose, and galactose, looks something like this:

Monosaccharides:	**Disaccharides:**
The simplest form of sugar	*2 monosaccharides bonded together*
Glucose (blood sugar)	Maltose (grain sugar) = glucose + glucose
Fructose (plant sugar)	Sucrose (cane, beet sugar) = glucose + fructose
Galactose (milk sugar)	Lactose (milk sugar) = glucose + galactose

Our culture is addicted to sucrose in many ways. What is usually listed in the food additives as sugar is some form of sucrose. Since sugar is excessive in the commercial food supply, and we know that sugar abuse is a problem, some food manufacturers are trying to obscure their listing of it as an ingredient. Vague labels such as, "evaporated cane juice" or "crystallized cane powder" are appearing on your favorite food products. It is just sugar.

Both sucrose and salt are the two most used commercial food ingredients. If you start seeing salt listed as "distilled sodium chloride" or "evaporated sea mineral," you know someone is attempting to veil something.

Refined sugar is problematic for the body because the minerals and fiber of the sugar cane or beet have been chemically stripped away. The refining produces a highly acidic producing chemical, one with many negative health effects. You know sugar is not great for you, but you take it in excess anyways—it is like a drug. Here are three things that are undisputed in the dietary frontlines, where there is often less agreement than discord:

1. Excess sugar consumption causes dental carries (cavities).
2. Excess sugar consumption is a significant factor in obesity.
3. People who have removed refined sugar from their diets have shown remarkable improvement in their health and wellness. Jack Lalanne, for example, America's first television health guru, whom I recall watching as a youngster (along with his German shepherd named Happy), attributes his robust health to his forsaking refined sugar and processed foods.[3] At 90 years, Jack is still going strong. May we all learn a few lessons from his example. (See segment on sugar in chapter 14.)

The Group Two collection contains carbohydrates that are long-chain assemblies of monosaccharides and disaccharides, known as polysaccharides or starch. These are commonly called complex carbohydrates because of the numerous groupings of simple sugars.

Three primary types of starches are (1) dietary starches (grains, roots, beans); (2) dietary fiber (carbohydrates that cannot be digested by human enzymes but can be by others in the animal kingdom); (3) glycogen (starch stored in your muscles and organs).

Starches are good sources of energy, especially corn, beans, and whole grains, but should not be eaten in excess. Part of the food combining guideline is to moderate, but not necessarily eliminate, starch intake,[4] especially past 49 years of age or with physical inactivity. (Refer to "Three Levels of Food Combining" in chapter 8.)

Recall that complex carbohydrates are simple sugars that are chained together. When the body breaks apart the sugar chains and uses them for fuel, the net result is sugar hitting the blood; the more starch you eat, the more this turns to sugar. This is what happens when you get "pasta intoxication" and feel very sleepy after the huge ravioli, potato gnocchi, and garlic bread feast. For diabetics, this is an extremely poor choice and could even be dangerous.

Usually both water and fiber occur in nature with carbohydrates. This helps slow down the rate at which the starch becomes glucose in the blood. The reason whole grains are steadily recommended is that the fiber of the husk and endosperm helps the body to efficiently process the starch and move it out of the gastrointestinal tract after assimilation. The fiber and water also help slow down the rate at which starch gets converted to blood sugar, minimizing, although not necessarily eliminating increased blood sugar spikes.

Things get thoroughly complicated when you mix too many different nutrients with a lot of starch (either in amount or in variety). All types of digestion chaos ensue, and it is possible that animal proteins will be on the deficient end of digestion, leaving you with meats that may ferment in the intestine. This is certainly a possibility with a person living with chronic constipation, a smoking habit, eating large amounts of refined and processed convenience foods, and having an inactive physical lifestyle. This is a true recipe for disease.

Desirable Starches:
- *Whole grains* (This means they have not been refined; they do not have the bran removed)
  - Naturally acid–forming: Brown rice, spelt, barley, oats, rye, corn
  - Naturally alkaline–forming: quinoa, millet, amaranth
- *Root Vegetables*

- Beets, carrots, ginger, potatoes, radishes, yams, sweet potatoes
- *Ground, stalk, or stem vegetables*
  - Artichokes, asparagus, bamboo shoots, broccoli, pumpkin, squash, turnips

Undesirable Starches:
- All refined bread products (that is, white bread)
- White rice, instant rice
- White potatoes in excess and especially without the peeling
- Any other intestinal clogging material (ICM)[5]

The Group Three collection of complex carbohydrates used to be called *roughage* but now goes by the less exertive name *dietary fiber*. There are two major types of fiber: soluble and insoluble.

Soluble fiber is fiber that dissolves in water. When you eat a plant, say an apple, it is the apple pulp that is the soluble fiber. These fibers form a gummy, jelly-like material when mixed with water in the intestines and are credited with lowering blood cholesterol levels and slowing the absorption of sugars into the blood, which is very beneficial to people with blood sugar imbalances, diabetes, and hypoglycemia. It is the soluble fiber that primarily produces methane and other gas byproducts of digestion, creating flatulence.

Insoluble fiber is the part of the plant, mostly the cell walls, which our digestive system cannot metabolize into energy. These fibers do not dissolve in water but rather absorb water like tiny sponges and help initiate peristalsis[6] in the intestinal tract. It is well known that many pathologies, from hemorrhoids and constipation to colon cancer, can be prevented by the regular intake of foods high in insoluble fiber, often called whole foods.

Type of Fiber	Benefits	Food Sources
Soluble	Decreases cholesterol in the blood; slows down glucose absorption	Apples Barley Broccoli Carrots Corn Dried beans Grapefruit Oat Bran Oats Oranges Potatoes Yams
Insoluble	Prevents constipation and the resultant hemorrhoids; may prevent colon cancer	Brown rice (rice bran) Flax seed meal Fruit & vegetable skins, peelings Green beans Green peas Nuts Seeds Wheat bran Whole-grain products

5

What Your Blood Recommends

They Say It's in the Blood[1]

THE FIGURATIVE USE OF BLOOD IS A WIDELY EMPLOYED LITERARY DE-vice crossing many generations and cultures. The Bible has a couple of hundred references to blood, starting with the Jewish myth of Cain and Abel. Cain kills Abel and right afterwards the "Lord said, 'What have you done? The voice of your brother's blood is crying to Me from the ground.'"[2] Even the ancient Semites knew there was something special and holy about blood millenia before microscopes would reveal some of blood's mysteries. Blood appears from Genesis to Revelations, from head to tail in the collection of books, as though the Bible itself were a body. The phrase "spilling of blood" is common throughout Semitic and Arabic folklore as a metaphor for death by murder or war, and can be found in both the Jewish Bible and the New Testament.

The Jewish observance of Passover is based on a story found in Exodus 12. The blood of a sacrificed goat or lamb smeared on the doorpost of an observant Israelite's home makes the Angel of Death "pass over" their dwelling (blood as a protective emblem).

The Christian tradition is founded upon the Eucharist: believers engage in an ancient rite to "drink the blood" of Christ (blood as a mystical medium).

Only John's Gospel has the story of Jesus turning water into wine at the wedding in Cana, as it certainly introduces John's version of Jesus' miraculous powers (blood as an indication of the awaited Messiah).

The ancient Persian myth of the prince–hero Esfandyar contains a crucial episode relating to blood (one reminiscent of the Greek myth of Achilles). Esfandyar is trying to cross a high mountain pass when a giant "Bird of Marvel" known as a *simurgh* tries to carry his chariot away. Esfandyar jumps to action, cutting the bird in two. The giant bird's blood covers him "from head to toe, making him invulnerable to any weapon." The hero instinctively closes his eyes when this deluge of blood happens (after all, wouldn't you?), which then makes only his eyes vulnerable to harm. Somehow the simurgh makes a remarkable recovery and tells the warrior Rostam to make a double–headed arrow and shoot for Esfandyar's eyes, his only place of susceptibility. Sure enough it works, and the hero dies tragically at the story's end.

Blood is a fascinating substance and a powerful mythic image throughout history. Modern science is still discovering much of the unrevealed configuration of blood, from numerous peptide combinations to viral activities.

But just what is blood, and what is it made of?

Blood is composed of a mixture of what is commonly called formed elements and a watery liquid called plasma. The formed elements consist of about 99.9% red blood cells (also known as erythrocytes or red cells), the most abundant blood cell and the constituent that gives blood its red appearance. The other .1% of the formed elements is a combination of platelets (which are crucial to the blood's ability to coagulate or clot when, for example, tissue is lacerated) and white blood cells. The blood plasma is composed of about 92% water, with the other 8% consisting of plasma proteins, electrolytes (specific mineral salts that conduct bioelectricity), and other organic properties.

The bottom line is this—everything relative to good health depends on the quality of the blood, which nourishes, transports, filters, and strengthens. Here are just a few crucial duties of blood:

1. Blood evens out your body temperature. When you exercise and become overheated, your blood absorbs the heat that is generated by your muscles and disperses it to other tissues. The excess

heat then becomes transferred across the skin's surface, and you sweat. If your body temperature is too low, then warm blood gets targeted towards the brain and temperature-sensitive organs (which is one reason you stay warmer with your head covered— about one third of your body temperature can be retained that way).

2. Blood is the defense against diseases. That hidden, rich red stream is a highway for white blood cells to remove wastes, toxins, and dead or damaged cells from the body. White blood cells are various elements that compose the immune system and create resistance against an assortment of pathogens. White blood cells travel from one place to another through the bloodstream. It is really quite a miracle how intelligent and efficient the body is in this way—all without your conscious awareness. Although most of the white blood cells are contained in the lymph fluid (think of it as clear blood that has its own designated highway through which to travel), the transporting capability of the blood is crucial to the effectiveness of white blood cells and robust immunity.

3. The plasma in the blood helps regulate the acidity and alkalinity of the fluid around your cells. Fluids continually circulate between the interstitial fluid (fluid that surrounds cells) and plasma; therefore, any notable alterations in the composition of the interstitial fluid rapidly affect the plasma. Your blood and the tissues that are supplied by blood have a sophisticated communication arrangement.

4. Last but not least, your blood is the superhighway for transporting metabolic wastes, hormones, nutrients, and dissolved gases throughout the body. Oxygen travels from the lungs to the peripheral tissues, and carbon dioxide goes from the tissues to the lungs. Nutrients from foods and vitamins stored in fat tissue and the liver are routinely transported through the bloodstream. Much of the cellular waste products are absorbed by the blood and taken to the kidneys or expelled through the lungs. There is a lot happening at any given moment in the blood.

Thanks to the Nobel Prize–winning scientist Karl Landsteiner, we have a system that recognizes four primary blood types. Interestingly, this crucial identification system has only been around since 1903.

Over three-fourths of the population has either A+ or O+ blood. The rarest blood type is AB, found in about one percent of the population.[3] The following is a small sampling of the global average:

Ethnicity	Type O %	Type A%	Type B%	Type AB%	% Rh factor +
African-American	49	27	20	4	85
Australian Aborigines	44	56	0	0	100
Caucasian	45	40	11	4	85
Chinese	42	27	25	6	100
Filipino	44	22	29	6	100
Hawaiian	46	46	5	3	100
Japanese	31	39	21	10	100
Korean	32	28	30	10	100
Native North Americans	79	16	4	<1	100
Native South Americans	100	0	0	0	100

Two important bits of knowledge for your insight into good health are these: (1) your blood type and (2) your metabolic dominance. Although somewhat related, they address different aspects of your unique metabolic/genetic configuration. Most researchers and holistic dieticians today will only loosely rely on blood type as a dietary guide, as they feel it is not infallible for a person's specific needs, but is more useful as a general starting point.

The short story of the relevance of your blood type to your diet goes something like this:

As a human species, we evolved (and are still evolving) in stages. As early *Homo sapiens* our dietary habits established certain biochemical predispositions in the tribe. We relied heavily on animal proteins for an extended period of time. As time evolved, we became an agrarian culture as we stayed in one place, cultivated plants, and domesticated wild animals. Our genetic blueprint therefore represents the accumulated lifestyle habits of our ancestors—both their strengths and weaknesses. Some people do well on meats, others on vegetables and grains, others still on some combination of the two.

Choosing foods based on your blood type provides insight into foods that you should avoid. A prime reason for many of the dietary restrictions cautioned against in this system is the presence of a substance in foods called lectin. Lectins are simply defined as proteins that specifically bind carbohydrates.[4] These substances are still being researched, and much is left to know about them. Lectins appear to agglutinate, or clump together, red blood cells, which may trigger a kind of allergic reaction in the body. If the right lectin comes in contact with the right receptor site in a cellular system, it could theoretically damage the cell, eventually compromising one's immunity. Blood typing nutrition is based on evolving research which speculates that certain foods act as a benefit or a detriment to your immune system, based on the lectins in a given food and your body's cellular reaction. Getting your diet in accord with your blood type may bolster your immune system, according to some advocates of this system.

Some researchers claim certain foods are high in lectins and are bad for everyone. The most commonly implicated foods are grains (especially wheat and wheat germ), legumes (including peanuts and soy-beans), dairy (especially the milk of grain-fed cows), and vegetables of the nightshade family (eggplant, peppers, potatoes, tomatoes).

The truth is, it all depends. Some people can eat these foods with no problem, and others can have significant reactions against them. There are many factors that influence how a person reacts unfavorably towards a lectin group.

Some ways of preparing the foods will mitigate the bioavailability of lectins. Sprouting grains, for example, reduces their lectin content. Fermenting appears to do the same with milk products. Much of the milk supply derived from cows has been substantially influenced by the inclusion of antibiotics, growth hormones, and many alterations in the cows' natural diet. There still is no successful substitution for fresh-growing, chlorophyll-rich, pesticide-free grass as a cow's ideal food. This clearly produces the best-quality milk. For some, even fermenting milk from grain-fed commercially raised cows may not be sufficient to reduce their allergic reactions to the milk.

Keep in mind as you read the following that it is the *quality* of the nutrient that is paramount—not all animals are raised in excellent conditions, and not all vegetables are grown in the most nutritious soil.

Type O Blood

The earliest evolutionary pattern is reflected in Type O blood, a genetic arrangement that dominates in most human bodies. This genetic predisposition promotes certain nutrients as favorable and others as distressing. If you are a Type O, the following are recommended:

- Eat meats, poultry, and seafood (all in moderate portion sizes, of course)
- Minimize your intake of dairy products, and if you are of African ancestry, eliminate all dairy. Some Asians do well on dairy, and some do not, so pay attention to how you feel with any given dairy product. Remember that whole dairy is almost always a better choice than the modified varieties.
- Oils are beneficial, the best being olive and flaxseed oils; canola,

cod liver, and sesame oils are your second choices. It is recommended that you avoid all other oils.

- Nuts and nut butters are a good vegetable protein for your blood type. The highest recommendation goes to almond butter and tahini (sesame seed butter), which are both commercially available. Be aware that you could still have a peanut allergy (which is technically a legume, not a nut), one of the most common food allergens.

- The bean and legume family is not the best food group for your blood type, but there are certain varieties that do better than others. Also, if you are of Asian ancestry, you have a favorable disposition towards legumes and beans and therefore a wider range of choices. Adzuki and pinto beans, as well as black-eyed peas, are most favorable; navy and kidney beans, as well as lentils, are least beneficial. Experiment and see what works best.

- Some cereals are recommended just as long as you avoid whole-wheat products (which is quite a challenge in most supermarket offerings). The "yes" column includes amaranth, barley, buck-wheat, kamut, millet, and spelt. The "no" column contains cornflakes, cornmeal, cream of wheat (or anything wheat like shredded wheat, wheat germ/bran, and so forth), Grape Nuts, and oat bran or oatmeal. Instant oatmeal is not good for anyone, especially Type Os.

- Have little to no grains (including bread) and pastas. If you really are longing for a pasta dish, you should try and locate rice flour, Jerusalem artichoke, or buckwheat pastas (or learn how to make them yourself). The standard durum semolina pastas are to be shunned by blood type Os, especially if you have insulin-dependant diabetes.

- Vegetables are required for type Os and should be eaten regularly, but there are certain varieties for which you should be very discriminating. Anything made with corn you should stay clear of, particularly if diabetes or obesity runs in your family. The nightshade vegetables (eggplant, potatoes) should also be avoided. Also, pass up any of the Brassica family of vegetables—

mustard greens, cauliflower, Brussels sprouts, and cabbage. The last bit of advice for Type Os, according to this system, is that certain microscopic molds in mushrooms and olives may trigger allergic reactions. It is advised that both of these foods be avoided, or at least pay close attention to how you feel after eating them. The good news is that Type Os and Type ABs can eat tomatoes; just choose the vine-ripened variety or get organic canned tomatoes, which are already ripe prior to canning.

- You can enjoy most fruits except blackberries, strawberries, oranges, and tangerines. Many type Os apparently have a strong reaction against coconut and coconut oils, so omit the Mai-tai when visiting the Tiki Lounge. Honeydew melon and cantaloupe are also not recommended on your shopping list. When it comes to fruit juices, the old standards of apple and orange juices are to be excluded from your pantry stockpiles, but any other juice not of previously proscribed fruits or vegetables is okay.

- Since Type Os tend to fall on the acidic side of the pH–base scale, it is recommended that they avoid some of the most commonly consumed beverages: coffee, black tea, hard alcohol, and all soft drinks. "What is left?" you may be asking. Beer is okay in small doses; just remember that if you are wanting to shed those extra pounds, too much Miller time might be a killer time. Green and herbal teas are suggested along with moderate amounts of red and white wine. Of course, there is always the excellent alkalizer of fresh lemon or lime juice in purified drinking water.

Type A Blood

The Type A blood signature evolved out of the Type O and results from a more agrarian biological development. Type As thrive on vegetarian cuisine, quite the contrast from Type Os, who need considerable animal protein. If you are a Type A, the following are recommended:

- Become a vegetarian. If this is a novel concept to you, it may require a transition over time in order to be successful—you cannot likely make the transition overnight. The first priority for you is to forsake all red meats, pork, and veal . . . yes, today . . . go ahead and empty the freezer and make your neighbors (who hopefully are Type Os) very happy with a surprise protein present. You will want to get to know how to prepare turkey and chicken dishes in your transition time and keep your portion sizes small (fist size or smaller). Those of Caucasian or African ancestry should get serious about limiting both portion size and frequency of consuming animal proteins. If you can make the transition within sixty days, it may be one of the most beneficial adjustments you make for your health—if sooner, so much the better. Since fish sources are getting more polluted with our intensifying industrial muscle, you will want to be selective in where you purchase you fish and seafood. There are some aquatic protein sources that are beneficial to Type As: carp, cod, grouper, mackerel, red snapper, trout, salmon, whitefish, and perch. Second in the ranking are the following fish: tuna, mahi–mahi, pike, sea bass, shark, snapper, sturgeon, swordfish, and yellowtail. You see, Type As can still enjoy a visit to the local sushi bar. Dr. D'Adamo also recommends that women with a history of breast cancer make snail a regular visitor at the table (perhaps accompanied with garlic and butter).[5] There seems to be a positive agglutinative effect with snail and mutated cells of Type As.

- If you are a lover of dairy products and have a Type A blood pattern, you have one of two choices: (1) Get a complete blood transfusion or (2) Eliminate most dairy. Since most of you will logically opt for the second choice, there is good news for you— some dairy products you can enjoy without too much regret. Since fermenting dairy helps break down the sugars that irritate the digestive tract of many Type As (and which consequently may weaken the immune system), much of the recommended dairy comes in an aged form. This gives you the opportunity to enjoy yogurt and kefir and the following cheeses: feta, goat cheese (and if you really want, goat milk), mozzarella, ricotta, and string cheese. Pay attention to how you feel eating the other dairy products, as they may not do well for you.

- Soy products are proliferating in the marketplace and are often suggested for Type As (for example, soy cheese and soy ice-cream) The central concern that you need to be aware of is that most of the soybeans grown in the U.S. are genetically modified. If you have access to soy products grown in Europe or Japan, you have a much better chance of their being GMO-free. Eggs are allowable; just obtain a good-quality egg from a free-range growth-hormone-free bird.

- Type As require very little fat consumption to maintain good health. A little good quality fat goes a long way for Type As, the best being olive oil and flaxseed oil. Since you cannot cook easily with flaxseed oil, you should get well acquainted with extra virgin olive oil. Canola oil is another option, but all other polyunsaturated vegetable oils should be avoided.

- When you take your red meat supply over to your neighbors tonight, ask them if they have any peanut butter, and make a trade. Since it is not beneficial for them but is for you, it makes a decent exchange. Nuts and seeds are an excellent protein and fat source for Type As, the only exceptions being Brazil nuts, cashews, and pistachios. Also, pumpkin and sesame seeds are an excellent choice, and there are many creative ways to incorporate them, as well as nut butters, into recipes.

- Type As do very well on beans and legumes and are encouraged to partake in them freely. The only restriction is that some beans have a lectin that increases insulin in the pancreas, which would not be favorable to diabetics or the obese. These would be garbanzo, navy, lima, and kidney beans. There are dozens of varieties of beans on the market, so there are diverse options.

- Most all whole-grain cereals should be favorable to Type As; however, there can be Type As who have a wheat gluten intolerance or allergy. If this is the case, avoid all wheat-based grain products and substitute with barley, oat, amaranth, buckwheat, or cornmeal. If you do not have a wheat sensitivity, all whole grains should be favorable. Try and buy (or make yourself) sprouted grain products, which are more nutritious and not agglutinating.

For everyone, the rule of thumb is to avoid all refined grains when possible, including white rice and white bread.

- Vegetables are your dietary staple. The only exceptions are peppers, which may aggravate your stomach, and olives (again, the mold in the fermentation). Tomatoes are not suitable because of their agglutinating property. This applies as well to white potatoes, yams, and cabbage. Otherwise, be creative and enjoy the fruits of the earth abundantly.

- Speaking of fruits, you have almost your pick of the litter. There are a few exceptions: avoid all tropical fruits including mango, papaya, and banana. The only tropical variety that does not generally interfere with Type A digestion is pineapple, whose abundance of the enzyme bromelain is music to your stomach's ears. Melons also can be problematic to the sensitive digestive system of Type As, as can many varieties of oranges. The other members of the citrus family should be welcome additions to your table—they are high in vitamin C and wholesomely alkalizing. For your juices, follow the same recommendations as above: no orange, papaya, coconut, or tomato juices.

- For your beverage choices, you get to be included in the lucky club that allows coffee consumption; just be careful about too much caffeine and remember that black is best. The number two choice is black coffee with a sweetener other than refined cane sugar, and the least desirable is coffee with any milk included. Green tea and moderate amounts of red and white wine can be beneficial. Avoid beers, sodas, hard alcohol, and black teas.

Type B Blood

You are fortunate with such an adaptable blood pattern. It seems that Type Bs branched off from Type Os to evolve into a more refined and versatile biological constitution. Whereas Type Bs have established a strong immunity against many of the common pathologies plaguing modern society (arteriosclerosis, cancers), they have likewise become vulnerable to the more uncommon varieties like chronic fatigue syndrome, irritable bowel syndrome, ALS, multiple sclerosis, and the like. Even with this slight vulnerability, in comparison to the other blood types, Type Bs are robust and adaptable, and this allows for a wide diversity in your food choices. If you are a Type B, the following are recommended:

- Eat red meat—lean red meat such as lamb, mutton, rabbit, and venison. Chicken is not a good choice for your blood type because of the detrimental effects of its inherent lectins upon your blood. You would be better off eating lean beef, buffalo meat (which is naturally leaner than beef), or turkey. You also get a wide variety of fish to choose from, with the exception of shellfish, which is not beneficial to your constitution.

- Dairy is indispensable for all Type Bs, with the exclusion of some people of African lineage who may have a residual lactose intolerance. Always pay attention to your body's messages after you eat. Eggs, cheeses, and milk products are well suited to your blood type, and—with the exception of an occasional allergy or food sensitivity—you should enjoy them heartily.

- Small amounts of quality fats taken regularly are very good for Type Bs, the best being olive oil, with flaxseed oil and cod liver oil being good second alternatives. It is advisable that you avoid all other polyunsaturated oils. Sesame oil, which is a staple for many Type Bs of Asian ancestry, is also recommended against although this oil has a very stable composition and is used widely throughout the world. Sesame oil, just like olive oil, contains antioxidant properties.

- Nuts and seeds are not the best food for Type Bs; however, in small amounts taken irregularly, almond and macadamia nut butters are usually tolerable. Most all other nuts and seeds are inconsistently beneficial to Type Bs.

- The bean and legume families are not as favorable to Type Bs as they are to other blood types. Black–eyed peas, lentils, garbanzo, and pinto beans are to be shunned, but kidney, lima, and navy beans are permissible.

- Cereals are a mixed bag for Type Bs: the beneficial varieties include spelt, oatmeal, and millet; the cereals to avoid are rye, amaranth, barley, wheat, buckwheat, and all corn products. As for bread products, avoid all wheat products and look for Essene or Ezekiel bread products found in many natural food stores. There are quality wheat-free and gluten-free breads on the market, along with brown rice and spelt breads. Rice is considered a neutral food for Type Bs. You can partake of semolina pastas in small amounts, which includes most commercial varieties of noodles. I recommend trying quinoa and brown rice as a grain substitute; they are versatile and easy to prepare.

- Type Bs get to enjoy the widest diversity available in the vegetable and fruit kingdoms. The exception is tomatoes, which neither Types A or B tolerate well. Corn and corn products and olives are also not advised. You do get to fancy mushrooms, the cabbage family, yams and potatoes—something the other blood types may be envious of. If you are a Type B with a fragile immune system, and prone to feeling cold, you should eat more dark leafy-greens, ginger, garlic, and onions to bolster your immunity and increase internal heat.

- Fruits are not very restricted, the exceptions being coconuts, rhubarb, pomegranates, and persimmons. This same unconstrained choice applies as well to juices, be they vegetable or fruit. As a Type B, you have a wide spectrum to choose from and enjoy.

- Your beverage choices are not too limited. Green teas are the superior drink for you, but black coffee and tea and the occasional glass of beer or wine should not be unfavorable to your constitution. Steer clear of hard alcohols and sodas of all assortments.

Blood Type AB

Type ABs possess the most unpredictable and puzzling constitution of all four. Being a hybrid of the A and B type, they assume the characteristics of both in varying degrees. This is the youngest of all the evolutionary types, being "less than a thousand years old [and] rare (2–5%

of the population)."[5] Of the four primary blood types, ABs need to pay closest attention to what foods work and do not work for their health and wellness. If you are a Type AB, the following are recommended:

- Meats are a tricky item for Type ABs to eat. You are genetically deficient in stomach acids needed to digest animal proteins, like your Type A relatives, but you need lean meats to help balance your nervous system and regulate your metabolism, like Type Bs. The solution is to moderate your consumption of animal meats, forsaking beef and pork in favor of lamb, turkey, and—most of all—fish and seafood. All of the seafood rules for Type As apply to your situation with these other specifications:

- Just as Type As, you should stay clear of sole and flounder. Also, avoid the following: anchovies, all bass, all shellfish, eel, frog, halibut, octopus, oysters, shrimp, and turtle.

- The recommended fish are tuna (just remember that mercury-free tuna supplies are getting more difficult to find), cod, grouper, mackerel, mahi–mahi, perch, pike, trout, red snapper, salmon (try and locate wild, not farm–raised), sardines (same problem with tuna applies to this fish), snail (which is very beneficial to Type As), and sturgeon.

- It is fortunate for you that your Type B gene governs when it comes to dairy. Type Bs have the widest freedom in the diversity of dairy products they can eat, and Type ABs get to benefit, as well. All fermented dairy is preferable (cottage cheese, yogurt, kefir, sour cream), along with eggs. Watch your portion size and keep your fat intake to a modest level—it is easy to overindulge with dairy and gain too much weight since dairy fat is a rich source of energy.

- The oils and fats recommended most for the AB Type are olive oil and ghee (clarified butter). If these are not available, then the next recommendations are canola and flaxseed oil. Avoid the other polyunsaturated oils.

- Beans and the legume family are advisable for Type ABs, the most desirable being lentils, red beans, pinto beans, navy beans, and soy beans. Type ABs are advised to minimize or eliminate their use of black-eyed peas, lima, fava, kidney, garbanzo, black, and adzuki beans.

- Cereals are favorable for Type ABs. If you are trying to shed those extra pounds, it is advisable not to eat wheat or corn products. The delicious grains of spelt, oat, quinoa, and millet are recommended for you to try. The same counsel applies to bread products—try wheat-free, Ezekiel, Essene, and soy flour breads. Rice is a favorable grain for your constitution; I recommend substituting brown rice for white rice and mixing brown and wild rice together for a nutty and enjoyable change of pace. Pastas should not be problematic for you; just keep the portion size to a reasonable amount (which would be about one fist size or one ladle scoop, which is way less than most standard servings).
- Vegetables are a necessary part of your dietary need. Type ABs have a wide diversity to choose from with a few exceptions: no corn products or peppers. This same unhindered approach applies to fruits. Just like Type As, you do not flourish on tropical fruits (except pineapple), so avoid them as well as oranges (and orange juice). You may also want to monitor your use of melons and see how a particular variety makes you feel afterwards. Grapefruit, lemons, and limes are desirable, as are grapes, figs, cherries, and kiwi.
- You have diversity in your beverage choices, the most essential being green and herbal teas. Coffee, beer, and wine are also fine for your Type AB constitution. Steer clear of black teas, hard alcohol, and all sodas.

Blood Type and Foods—Quick-Look Chart[1]

Blood Type O

Meats
Yes—3 days a week.

Animal proteins work well for you—find a good organically raised source.

Lean varieties are best (stay clear of fatty pork, goose, etc.).

You need only a *small amount* at a meal—the size of your fist or smaller—especially if you are trying to lose weight.

Make sure you have fresh vegetables at every meal. The more weight you want to shed, the greater your vegetable portions to meat.

Fish & Seafood
Yes—4 days a week.

Fish and seafood are an excellent choice for your blood type. Make sure the water source from which the fish come is unpolluted.

Dairy & Eggs
Only in small amounts.

Dairy is not a great choice for you (especially those of African heritage). Choose the low-fat (skim) varieties but do not buy foods with fat substitutes; you are better with real fat in small amounts.

Small amounts of organic butter and skim cheese on an occasional basis should work for you.

Try soy cheese and milk. There are many soy products on the market that mimic meat proteins in a convincing way.

Beans & Legumes
Only in small amounts.

Although not ideal for you, there are a few varieties that should be acceptable to your digestion: black-eyed peas, pinto and adzuki beans, the latter of which are high in protein.

Fats
Yes, in moderation.

Since Type Os tend to exhibit cardiovascular pathologies, good quality fats (no fat substitutes, hydrogenated oils, etc.) taken on a moderate basis can be beneficial if accompanied by regular exercise.

Get to like extra-virgin olive oil and flaxseed oil. Use small amounts of sesame and canola oils and avoid the other polyunsaturated oils.

Blood Type and Foods—Quick-Look Chart

Blood Type O

Cereals/Grains
Not recommended.

Processed cereals are a no-no.

Many Type Os have a wheat intolerance, so it is advisable that you eliminate all wheat and wheat products (which is about 95% of the commercial breads and bread products.)

Try experimenting with alternative grain foods: gluten-free breads, soy and amaranth cereals and pastas, whole rye and spelt breads, etc.

When you do choose grains, eat whole grains and in portions not exceeding your cupped palm.

Vegetables & Fruits
Yes—7 days a week.

Not so beneficial:
Vegetables
- corn, white potatoes (yams and sweet potatoes are better), eggplant, cabbage, Brussels sprouts, mustard greens, cauliflower, mushrooms.

Fruit
- melons
- oranges & tangerines
- strawberries and blackberries

Beneficial:
Vegetables
- dark leafy-greens (chard, kale, spinach, broccoli, collard and dandelion greens, etc.)
- vine-ripened tomatoes (or canned)
- garlic and onions
- okra
- all other vegetables

Fruit
- plums, prunes, figs, dates
- mango, papaya, kiwi
- apples
- grapes

Blood Type and Foods—Quick-Look Chart
Blood Type A

Meats
Not Recommended.

Try to make fish and seafood your primary meat sources. Your system is most comfortable as a vegetarian.

Fish & Seafood
Yes—2-4 days a week.

The main food recommendations are carp, cod, grouper, mackerel, monkfish, red snapper, salmon, sardines, trout, snails.
It is advisable that you minimize or avoid all other fish and seafood (or have very small amounts.)

Dairy & Eggs
Not recommended, unless in a fermented form.

Organic eggs are suitable in small amounts. The ideal cooking method is poaching.

Fermented dairy (organic is advisable): yogurt, kefir, cottage cheese, sour cream, cheese.

Soy, rice, and goat milks are acceptable surrogates.

Beans & Legumes
Yes—3-5 days a week.

If you have diabetes or obesity it is advisable that you avoid kidney, lima, navy, and garbanzo beans. Otherwise, all beans and legumes should prove favorable to you (not withstanding an individual's food allergy, with peanuts being a very common food allergen.)

Fats
Yes, in moderation.

Type As need a small amount of good-quality fats to do well.

Your number one choice is olive oil, followed in order of preference by flaxseed oil, canola oil, and cod liver oil.

Nuts and seeds are a good protein-fat combination, so enjoy them abundantly.

Blood Type and Foods—Quick-Look Chart
Blood Type A

Cereals/Grains
Yes—5-7 days a week.

Avoid instant or processed cereals in favor of whole grain varieties.

Some good choices are amaranth, buckwheat, barley, kamut, millet, oats, spelt, and quinoa.

If you have a respiratory condition, it is advisable that you avoid wheat and wheat products.

Vegetables & Fruits
Yes—7 days a week.

Vegetables are your dietary staple.

Here are a few of the least recommended vegetables for your type: cabbage, eggplant, mushrooms, olives, peppers (all), white and sweet potatoes, and tomatoes.

Soy products are advisable, as well as broccoli, beets, collard and dandelion greens (along with all the dark leafy-greens), garlic and onions, pumpkin, squash, bean sprouts, turnips, parsnips, cucumber, and zucchini.

Anything not on the avoid list: Have at it, and bon appetit!

Most all fruits are beneficial with the possible exception of tropical fruits (mango, papaya, starfruit, etc.), melons, oranges and tangerines, bananas and plantains, and coconut.

Blood Type and Foods—Quick-Look Chart
Blood Type B

Meats
Yes, except for red meat and chicken.

Seafood is preferable, but you can have moderate amounts of lamb, venison, buffalo, turkey, and any game birds.

Fish & Seafood
Yes—3-5 days a week.

Avoid all shellfish in favor of cold-water fishes like salmon, sturgeon, mahi-mahi, trout, halibut, mackerel, and snapper.

Caviar is a satisfactory food for your Type.

Dairy & Eggs
Yes—3-5 days a week.

If you are of African or Asian ancestry, you may have a more difficult time digesting dairy products; experiment and see. Eating fermented dairy may alleviate many of the associated problems.

Type Bs have the greatest choice of selection when it comes to enjoying dairy products.

Beans & Legumes
Yes, in moderation.

Unless you have a diabetic or obese condition, you should be able to enjoy these foods 1-2 days a week, especially kidney, lima, navy, and soy beans.

Fats
Yes, in moderation.

Olive oil is preferable; ghee (clarified butter) and flaxseed oils are reasonably good for you. It is advisable that you stay clear of the other oils.

Blood Type and Foods—Quick-Look Chart
Blood Type B

Cereals/Grains
Yes—2-3 days a week.

Whole grains are the key. Try mixing whole grains with beans for a hearty complete protein.

The preferred cereals are millet, oats, rice, spelt, and quinoa.

Not advisable are rye, wheat and corn (if you are diabetic or obese), and barley.

Vegetables & Fruits
Yes—7 days a week.

There are only a few vegetables that you should avoid: tomatoes, corn, olives, radishes, and artichokes.

The rest of nature's cornucopia you can enjoy abundantly.

Blood Type and Foods—Quick-Look Chart
Blood Type AB

Meats
Yes, in moderation; no red meat or poultry.

It is advisable that fish and seafood constitute a large part of your animal protein.

Fish & Seafood
Yes—3-5 days a week.

Depending on the genetics of the A-type or B-type dominance, you may not do well with shellfish; experiment and see. Cold-water fish that should benefit you: albacore tuna, cod, mackerel, mahi-mahi, perch, pike, trout, salmon, snail, and sturgeon.

Dairy & Eggs
Yes—2-3 days a week.

If you have symptoms of excess mucus (ear infections, sinusitis, respiratory trouble), you should eliminate dairy until you bolster your immunity. Otherwise, these foods should be helpful in modest amounts for Type ABs.

Beans & Legumes
Yes, depending on the variety.

Stick with the following: navy, pinto, and red beans. You can also enjoy lentils in all varieties.

It is recommended that you avoid the following: adzuki, black, fava, garbanzo, kidney, and lima beans, as well as black-eyed peas.

Fats
Yes, in moderation.

Olive oil is preferable; ghee (clarified butter) and flaxseed oils are reasonably good for you. Stay clear of the other oils.

Blood Type and Foods—Quick-Look Chart
Blood Type AB

Cereals/Grains
Yes—2-3 days a week.

The most favorable are millet, quinoa, oat, rice, and spelt.

If you are trying to lose weight or have a respiratory condition, stay clear of wheat and wheat products.

Vegetables & Fruits
Yes—7 days a week.

All the produce beneficial to A and B types works for you, as well. You are advised to avoid only the following: corn and corn products, tomatoes, olives, and peppers (all).

6

What Your Genes Recommend– Metabolic Typing

THE WAY YOUR BODY TURNS FOOD INTO ENERGY AND TISSUE IS A highly individualized process. Your genes set the template, but other factors, such as environment and disease, alter how you function within that template.

It has taken tens of thousands of years for humans to develop specific dietary requirements. Several factors establish predispositions in genetic inheritance. These various factors influence nutrient digestion in response to many dynamic aspects: habitat and lifestyle, climate, geographical terrain, quality of vegetation, and naturally occurring food supplies. Different tribes have evolved in ways that make certain foods more favorable than others. The blood typing scheme is a good place to start to understand what basically works and what does not: do you function best on proteins or complex carbs? The next step is to understand just how you metabolize foods: are you oxidative- or autonomic-dominant? This helps you get more specific about your particular needs.

It is sensible to start with what your particular tribe has eaten in its development. For example, inhabitants of cold northern regions of the world have historically depended very heavily on animal protein as a sustaining nutrient, merely because that's the principal food source available in frigid climates; not too many edible plants can survive in freezing weather. As a result, northerners have developed different nutritional requirements from people of equatorial and sub-tropical regions, where there is a wide variety of vegetation year-round.

During the 1930s, an adroit dentist from Cleveland, Ohio, named Weston Price, with pragmatic scientific common sense, confirmed this theory in some remarkable ways. He journeyed around the world in search of indigenous populations who had not yet met the ill fate of humans consuming post-industrial cuisine. He completed this experiment at the perfect time—just before the oblivious tendrils of technology and politics would decimate these people's traditional foods and eventually many of the tribes themselves. Dr. Price studied the diet and health of some twelve major regions and many subcultures within those regions. What he discovered is extraordinary for the 1930s and quite prophetic for today. A few of his principal conclusions were these:

1. Different people eat different things depending on where they are on the planet. Even though there were common strands among them, the food sources of various indigenous people were diverse, being contingent on climate, terrain, and availability, as well as tradition.

2. There are certain foods that one's genetic blueprint reacts favorably towards. The indigenous communities that followed their natural ancestral diets were thoroughly healthy, with very low incidents of dental carries (cavities) and strong, symmetrical bone structure of the face and body.

3. The people who strayed from their ancestral diet acquired health deterioration, often within one generation. The body's immunity declined, dental carries and weak and misshapen bones developed, behavioral problems emerged, and other pathologies soon followed. There are certain foods that one's genetic and biochemical inclination reacts unfavorably towards.

4. Some of the most common ailments occurred as a result of the newer foods that were being consumed by the people, foods that reached them through the advent of technology. Refined sugar, jams, white breads and bread products, processed cereals, canned vegetables (in place of fresh), confections, sweetened beverages, chocolate, and other modern products were noted as key to dietary imbalance. Today, the worrisome products are laden with

refined sugar, mutated (hydrogenated) fats, and genetically modified organisms.

5. When it comes to food, old-fashioned is often superior. Beware of
    excessive or habitual consumption of refined, sweetened, and
    processed food items. If it comes from Mother Nature, in a natu-
    ral form, it is the superior choice. Straying too far from Nature's
    format always incurs a heavy toll.

What we can gain from Dr. Price's work is that there is not a single
diet equally applicable for everyone, not a one-size-fits-all nutrition
scheme for the globe, although there are definitely foods that work
better than others.

We are a highly adaptive species, but there are limits to what we can
change and how fast we can change it; diet is but one example of this.
People eat whatever they locate regionally or what the climate will allow to be successfully cultivated. We can adapt to many types of regional foods, but we do not do well with synthetic materials in our food
supply, or with natural products that get refined, mutated, or otherwise
scientifically mutilated.

The indigenous people Dr. Price studied who stayed with their traditional foods were dramatically healthier then the same clan members
who became dependent upon modernized foods. The Eskimo families
or African Masai tribes could not endure long on fruit pies, soda, and
fast-food cuisine. The skyrocketing diabetes and heart disease rates
within Native American reservations and African-American communities should be alarming enough to prompt the question "What is not
working?" Asian communities, once the paragons of good health and
longevity but now adopting fast-food fare as a nutritional habit, are
seeing the same health complaints so prolific in the West. This should
be enough to ask the question "What is not working?"

In the 1930s, Dr. Price was already recording these changes. Dr. Price
documented "dental arch deformities . . . crooked teeth . . . narrow nostrils . . . changed facial form . . . " in the first generation to "have adopted
the white man's foods."[1]

We need to see foods in terms of their relative feasibility. If meat is
basically "bad" food, then we should examine the robust health of the

Inuit people (the Eskimos) who consume large amounts of animal meats, fish eggs, and seal oil. This also applies to the native inhabitants of the South Sea Islands, Micronesia, and the coastal indigenous people of Peru: animal meats and meat products are a central part of their traditional diets. We could add the Australian Aborigines and Native American Indians to that list and keep adding. Meats, in their natural unprocessed forms, are a beneficial dietary staple for these peoples.

Carbohydrates are not inherently problematic either. Just study the Quichua people of Peru's Andes Mountains, descendants of the Aztecs, whose high intake of starches has nourished the people for millennia. There are many other tribes who thrive on a whole grain and vegetable diet and whose genetic propensity is favorably disposed to quality non-processed carbohydrates.

If dairy is the main culprit of poor nutrition, then examine the Swiss, whose ancestral diet is established largely on dairy and whole rye, or the African Masai, who drink raw blood and milk mixed together. This also applies to the mountain inhabitants of the Himalayan regions: quality whole dairy products are central to their traditional diets.

Metabolic typing is the culmination of the work of many innovative doctors and pioneering researchers. This individualized understanding of our nutritional needs has developed over two and a half decades of research and clinical experience.

This dietary system is very compatible with and complimentary to dietary blood typing, analyzing the main metabolic indicators of the body to examine how a given person is utilizing nutrients. It is a more specified version of the blood typing system. Metabolic typing practitioners consider blood type as one of the main criteria in their analysis scheme.

Just as an automobile engine is designed to run on a certain type of fuel, gasoline or diesel, hydrogen or ethanol, we, too, have certain fuel inclinations that serve us optimally. Some people have a tendency to run best on proteins and fats, and others do best on carbohydrates. If you were to force diesel into a gas engine, or proteins into a carbohydrate–dominant person, problems would soon occur.

In the same manner, our bodies have biological requirements for particular kinds of foods and a certain nutritional equilibrium to maintain in order to be the most healthful. When we honor our natural fuel needs, we feel better and function optimally.

A multitude of complaints could accompany poor dietary choices, from weakness, low blood sugar, and fatigue to headaches, body aches, constipation, and irritability.

Some metabolic typing practitioners believe that chronic dietary negligence can contribute to more severe problems, from arthritis to neurological troubles. Of course, there is not just one factor involved in the progression of a serious pathology but a series of problems that accumulate without adequate resolution. Fatiguing your immune system from a diet inappropriate to your biologic needs could be a significant factor in the chain of progression.

Paying close attention to how your body feels with certain nutrients is crucial to understanding what foods work and what foods do not. Just because you have always eaten a certain food, or your family did, is not an indicator for continuing to eat it. Your parents may have had problems with a certain food that they did not convey, or the quality of the food product in question may have deteriorated through mass production. The key for you is to pay attention.

For a person who has a metabolic temperament that leans to the acidic, eating acid–producing foods will be counterproductive and cause distress. The same acid–producing food will be welcomed by the system of a person who is leaning to the alkaline side of the scale, resulting in better energy levels, mental clarity, and efficient digestion.

There are a multitude of diets in the mainstream, all promoting one certain way that will work well for everyone. Just through random chance, a person who is protein dominant could be chosen to participate in a high–protein diet and do well. The opposite would occur if a carb-dominant person were subjected to the same diet. In any given application of a certain diet there will be successes and failures, but eating in accord with your body's metabolic dominance shows consistently positive results.

Metabolic typing is based on the most fundamental rule of biology: every person is unique and needs to be treated as such. One size does not fit all in nature, in philosophy, or in health—there are many gray areas. The fact that certain foods work for me and do not for you is attributed to biochemical individuality—not the food itself. This happens in allopathic medicine with medications, doses, frequency, and other factors. It is equally applicable in nutrition.

The ancient physicians recognized that the same disease could be arrived at in many different ways. If the disease is treated but not the person, the chances of truly eradicating the cause or causes is haphazard at best. Metabolic typing addresses the individual's uniqueness, just as medicine once did and now is starting to again. We can hope that the modern medical system continues to learn from its mistakes and return to this ancient approach of treating the patient and not the pathology.

Just as a fireman cannot stop an inferno until he knows from where it is originating and from what cause, a medical specialist cannot treat a pathology until she knows how the patient arrived at this state and what factors were involved. Metabolic typing addresses this issue on a nutritional level by working with how *your* body processes various foods.

There are some well–intentioned people who have read about the virtues of an all–vegetarian diet and decided to adhere to this for the sake of their health. When they discover that they cannot sustain themselves on this regimen without feeling fatigued, foggy–minded, and lifeless, they shrink into themselves with depression, thinking perhaps that they are "just too unhealthy to eat healthy." The problem is not the nutrient; it is the approach that is not right for them. When they eat according to both their blood type dominance and their metabolic strength, their good health has a chance to return.

Portion size is a significant factor no matter what nutritional road you follow, and it is even more important if you are overeating the wrong nutrients for your metabolism. If you at least overeat the right nutrients, your body can recover more efficiently. Of course, the best plan is to eat the right amount of the right nutrients that work specifically for you. If you were to take a simple calorie reduction approach, you could be both needlessly starving yourself and introducing the inappropriate fuel for your body. What a mess.

Some people reduce calories and actually gain weight. How is that for confusing? If your body does not have the right fuel, you may actually trigger a craving response, producing a slingshot effect in the opposite direction. Just watch how the misguided protein–dominant person who is forcing himself to be a vegetarian slingshots into the local burger joint and dives face first into the double cheeseburger or two. Calorie reduction is not the answer, as much as eating the right amount of foods appropriate to your biochemical individuality: putting the right amount of diesel fuel in a diesel engine.

The Basic Plan

People fall into a few broad categories in metabolic typing. The type depends on what your body prefers for fuel and how it does it.

It is thought that the ideal blood pH is 7.46, which is leaning a bit to the alkaline side. There are two main categories of metabolizers: oxidizers and autonomics.

The oxidizers lean either to the fast or slow side. If you are a fast oxidizer, you burn up fuel quickly (which is oxidation), have a naturally acidic system (your blood wants to naturally dip to the acid side of 7.46), and you need to focus on eating proteins and fats to slow down your quick burn rate. Small amounts of proteins and fats taken at regular intervals work well for fast oxidizers.

As a slow oxidizer, you burn fuel slowly, have a naturally alkaline system, and need to focus on taking complex carbohydrates while minimizing, but not eliminating, your protein and fat intake. The amount of reduction you will make in proteins and fats will depend on just how extreme a slow oxidizer you are. This system is dynamic and changes with time. You may need to start out with very little proteins and fats and eventually, as your body adjusts, gradually add these nutrients back into your diet.

Autonomics will share food groups with the oxidizers but for different reasons. Recall that the autonomic nervous system is divided into two aspects: sympathetic (fight or flight) and parasympathetic (rest and digest).

If your nervous system sets the metabolic dominance in your body (instead of the cellular oxidation rate), you are a sympathetic type. If it is the sympathetic branch, you will share the same foods with slow oxi-dizers: more complex carbs and fewer proteins and fats. Sympathetics lean towards the acidic and need to have their parasympathetic aspect emphasized to keep them balanced. Sympathetics may be considered hyper personalities: on the go, easily sweating, fast talkers, lean, insom-niacs, with possible digestion problems.

Parasympathetics are just the opposite: they are slower, more delib-erate types, usually more short and stocky, have laid–back personalities, and tend toward low blood pressure. This type needs proteins and fats and fewer complex carbs. They are slower at burning fuel and need to have their alkaline systems balanced with the acidic benefits of proteins and fats, the same as the fast oxidizer.

7

Food Combining Rudiments

MOST OF THE EARLIEST INFORMATION WE HAVE REGARDING FOOD combining in the twentieth century traces back to the readings of Edgar Cayce and the work of Dr. Herbert Shelton and Dr. William Howard Hay. The two food combining philosophies, that of the doctors and that of Mr. Cayce, were simultaneously developed in the 1930s. Since Mr. Cayce appears to have accessed information based on tapping into a collective thought pool, the *collective unconscious* as Carl Jung penned it, perhaps he was intuitively accessing the work of the doctors as it was being developed. Although there are slight discrepancies when one compares the two food combining prescriptions, there are many areas that are in accord. Perhaps we can attribute slight incongruities to Mr. Cayce's ability to be very specific about a person's constitution. What may have worked for one person, or for most people, would not have been advisable for the particular person for whom the reading was given. It is similar to the traditional Asian medical systems (China, Tibet, et al); a different remedy is given based on *why* the person has a pathology. The same pathology may have five slightly different treatments for five different people. This is at odds with the post–industrial method of basically treating the pathology and not the person.

Here are some general food combining agreements that everyone can benefit from:
- Do not have more than two starches per meal. This is quite at

odds with the basic American meal, during which pasta, bread, potatoes, corn, and pie are often eaten at the same sitting. Pick just *two* and eat them in moderate quantities. Ahhhh . . . discipline is good.

NEWS:
May 9, 2002—**A diet high in starchy foods such as potatoes, rice, and white bread may increase the risk of pancreatic cancer in women who are overweight and sedentary, according to a new study by Dana-Farber Cancer Institute, Brigham and Women's Hospital and Harvard School of Public Health researchers.**[1]

- Eat citrus and melon by themselves. They interfere with the digestion of all other nutrients. By themselves, they are a good source of vitamins.
- Do not drink orange juice and milk at the same sitting; pick one or the other. As a matter of fact, milk—if you insist on taking it—is best taken with no other nutrients. Think about it; what else is a baby mammal going to eat other than mother's breast milk when feeding? Milk is a high fat/protein food perfect for babies. Mr. Cayce did recommend that some people drink cow's milk, but it is safe to recommend that unless in a fermented[2] and organic form, it is best to stay clear of it after you get your first set of teeth. If you insist on taking milk, you would do better to find goat's milk, as it is closer in composition to human milk than the bovine variety.
- Do not mix shellfish with any kind of alcohol. As it turns out, alcohols generally do not mix well with many nutrients, but especially not with shellfish. The old oysters and whiskey item is not the best menu choice when considering good food combining. Although, if you have enough of the latter item, you will probably not care.
- According to Mr. Cayce, meat with potatoes is preferable to meat

with breads. So, say farewell to sandwiches and meat pizzas. However, the recommendation was "not [to] eat great quantities of
starch with proteins or meats . . . "[3] Small amounts of starch are
not problematic for most; just chew it very well. Remember that
starches turn into sugars in the body. Sure, it looks like a harmless baked potato, but after digestion it becomes the equivalent of
2½ chocolate bars, relative to blood sugar.

- Tomatoes should be vine-ripened. It is best to eat them either
  alone and plain, with a little salt, or in a salad with green lettuce.
  Do not eat them unripe, with sugars or with any vinegars, which
  may lead to hyperacidity.
- No fried foods of any kind (good luck with that in the Southern
  states) and especially not fried potatoes. If you must indulge, less
  is more!
- Lettuce, celery, and carrots together (assuming they are organically grown) were recommended by Mr. Cayce to " . . . maintain
  such a condition as to immunize a person."[4] Think of it as a natural inoculation to boost the body's defenses. Regular salads would
  cover this. Fresh salads have many benefits; the more veggies, the
  better.
- Stay clear of soft drinks. The extra phosphoric acid and carbon-
  ation in the body is not seen as beneficial in any way. The Cola
  syrup, by itself without carbonated water added, was recommended as " . . . [aiding] in purifying the kidney and activity and
  bladder."[5] Carbonated water was not recommended.[6]
- Eat fresh, locally grown produce as "Shipped vegetables are never
  very good."[7]
- Moderate consumption of alcohol, especially in the evenings, was
  recommended as " . . . well for most bodies"[8] Cayce recommended
  red wine in the "late afternoon with black or brown bread,"[9] but
  not taken with meals. There is plenty of research to show that
  reasonable amounts of wine have an LDL-cholesterol-lowering
  and antioxidant effect. Because of the high sugar content in wine,
  it is best not to drink with a full stomach. One and a half to two
  hours after a meal is ideal.

- Do not use aluminum cookware. " . . . [foods] which are acid[ic] will take particles of aluminum into the body."[10] Cayce especially advised against putting " . . . certain fruits, or tomatoes, or cabbage"[11] into aluminum cookware. Read the label on your commercial deodorants; they often use an aluminum compound in the ingredients. What to use in place of aluminum cookware? Stainless steel and enamel instead.
- Pass on the instant oatmeal, " . . . [which] isn't good for anyone,"[12] in favor of the steel cut oats, which Cayce recommended in numerous readings. You can soak steel cut oats overnight to reduce the cooking time. All the whole grains are good foods. Try spelt, quinoa, millet, amaranth, rye, and barley.
- Do not mix proteins with sweets.[13] It is best to have meats without a sweetened sauce, jellies, or the like.
- Soy milk is recommended only to people who have very physical activities and are fire–types—active, hyper, with quick metabolisms. For people who spend much of the day doing mental work, taking soymilk, " . . . would not be so well."[14] Most of the Asian countries that are esteemed as paragons of soybean's virtues actually ferment the soybean. The results are foods such as tempeh and miso. Although a protein–rich legume, soy is recommended only occasionally and in a fermented form. Another complication is that soy is one of the most widely genetically modified crops in the U.S. There is an extensive controversy over the long–term safety of genetically modified organisms (GMOs) in our food supply.

Food Combining—Quick-View Chart (Based on the Edgar Cayce Health Readings)			
Food	**Goes well with . . .**	**A so-so combination with . . .** [1]	**Goes poorly with . . .**
Meat The most recommended meats are "fish, fowl, and lamb" and beef juice without the bulk.[2]	Vegetables and fats	Potatoes (breads are considered worse)	Starches, simple sugars (including fruit), and other meats[3]
Milk[4]	Nothing	Whole-grain breads	Citrus, meat, alcohol
Starches	Fats	Vegetables	Other starches, simple sugars, meat
Vegetables	Meats, fats, other vegetables	Starches	Simple sugars
Fruit[5] (not counting citrus, apples, and melons)	Water	Whole-grain breads, leafy vegetables (not roots), fats	Meats, refined starches
Citrus Fruits	Water	Whole-grain breads	Any dairy, meats, vegetables, other fruits, refined starches[6]
Melons	Water	Nothing	Everything
Apples[7] (raw)	Nothing	Nothing	Everything
Simple sugars	Nothing	Nothing	Everything

8

Three Levels of Food Combining

SINCE PEOPLE FUNCTION AT VARIOUS DEGREES OF WELLNESS, WE CAN break down food combining into three major categories to customize the approach. Note that with all three food–combining recommendations there are many gray areas to consider. You will have to customize these recommendations in accord with your blood and metabolic type to get optimal results. Within the following three categories you can find a starting place to adapt food combining to your particular health situation. All the general food–combining principles are applicable with the following as addendums.

Level #1: **Robust**

This is a plan for someone operating at an optimal wellness level.

The overview:

(A person can be any one, or combination, of the following.)

- Under 35 years old
- No major health complications (immune system is robust)
- Physically active (nothing significantly impeding their activities)
- Non–smoker and non–drinker (or very light social drinker)
- Basically within a normal height to weight ratio

The fundamental plan:
- Eat approximately 25% (by meal's weight) raw and/or green foods twice weekly.
- Soy products (fermented and non–GMO varieties are preferred) can be taken as long as physical activities are vigorous.
- Three starches are allowable per meal, twice a week. With starches, portion control is crucial. If your physical activity is less, your starch intake should be decreased.
- Combining fruits and vegetables should not pose a problem (except for tomato and melon, which are best eaten alone).
- Eat fruit 30 to 40 minutes after a meal of starch and fat; 60–90 minutes after animal proteins.
- Eat only minimal amounts of protein–starch combinations; root starches are preferable to grains when taken with animal proteins.[1]
- Unless there is a family history of heart disease or obesity, quality fats can be eaten plentifully. The premium choices are olive oil, canola oil, sesame oil, avocado, and organic ghee. If you become less physically active, reduce your fat intake.

Level #2: Transitional

This is a plan for someone operating at a moderately compromised wellness level.

The overview:

(A person can be any one, or combination, of the following.)

- Between 35 and 49 years of age
- Some minor health complications
- Activity level is moderate to minimal
- Some smoking and/or some alcohol usage
- Daily drug usage
- Energy levels are erratic, inconsistent, uneven

The fundamental plan:
- Eat approximately 50% (by meal weight) raw and/or green foods three times weekly.
- Take soy products only in fermented form, twice weekly.
- No more than two non-refined, unprocessed starches at any meal. Keep starch portions no bigger than the size of your cupped palm.
- Eat fruits and vegetables at separate meals.
- Eat fruit at the end of a meal of starch and fat; wait *at least* 40 minutes after the meal to enjoy the fruit.
- Keep meat consumption to a minimum: no more than half the size of your fist for a serving. Wild game and fish are the preferred animal proteins.[2]
- Try introducing more legume and whole-grain combinations, even in place of animal proteins, if that works for your system.
- Eat fats moderately. They should be of excellent quality. The premium choices are olive oil, canola oil, sesame oil, avocado, and organic butter or ghee. For Level 2 functioning, keep these fat portions the size of your thumbprint or smaller at any given meal. A little fat goes a long way.
- Drink at least one liter of purified water daily; 50% of this could include herbal tea (½ liter).

Level #3: **Declension**

This is a plan for someone operating at a considerably compromised wellness level. The overview:
(A person can be any one, or combination, of the following.)

- Past 50 years of age
- Notable health complications
- Activity level is very low to none (invalid)
- Recovering from surgery or a major medical intervention
- Daily multiple-drugs usage
- Recreational drug or alcohol addiction, or in recovery

The fundamental plan:

- Eat approximately 25% (by meal weight) raw and/or green foods *five* times weekly.
- Take soy products in fermented form, only once weekly.
- Eat only *one* starch per meal.[3]
- Eat fruits and vegetables at separate meals.
- Eat fruit at the end of a meal of starch and fat; wait at least 60 minutes after the meal to take the fruit.
- Try introducing more legume and whole-grain combinations in substitution for meat dishes.
- Eat fats moderately. They should be of good quality. The premium choices are olive oil, canola oil, sesame oil, avocado, and organic butter.
- Dietary calcium can be increased through the regular intake of yogurt, buttermilk, collard greens, fresh parsley, kale, and Swiss chard. Also, the herb shavegrass (horsetail) is quite high in minerals, including calcium. There are numerous calcium-phosphorus-magnesium supplements on the market.[4]
- You should supplement your diet with bran: oat bran, wheat bran, flax seed meal, and so forth. Always drink extra water when you take extra bran. You can add bran to many foods such as sauces, stews, and cereals without significantly altering their flavor.
- Drink at least one liter of purified water a day; 50% of this could include herbal tea (½ liter).

9

Sacred Ideas of Fasting

TRADITIONALLY, FASTS HAVE BEEN A PART OF RELIGIOUS OBSERVANCE and in modern times have been a form of sociopolitical protest. Food is a sign of power and abundance, wealth and affluence. In ancient Mesopotamia, the Assyrian priests ruled the granaries, giving them considerable social leverage. You can even examine the food–power relationship at work in reading the composition of the infamous nineteenth century abolitionist Frederick Douglass. In Douglass' *Narrative*, he describes the condition of slaves in Maryland in the 1830s, where controlling food was central in manipulating a slave's disempowerment:

> "We were not regularly allowanced. Our food was coarse corn meal boiled. This was called mush. It was put into a large wooden tray or trough and set down upon the ground. The children were then called, like so many pigs, and like so many pigs they would come and devour the mush; some with oyster-shells, others with pieces of shingle, some with naked hands, and none with spoons. He that ate fastest got most; he that was strongest secured the best place; and few left the trough satisfied."[1]

Religious traditions worldwide present dietary restrictions as a central tenet of religious compliance. Contrary to the ruthlessness of diet restrictions in pre–Civil–War slavery, these dietary restrictions are intended to be physically and spiritually empowering,

In Jewish customs, it is the Laws of Kashrut, culled largely from Leviticus 11 (but also found in Exodus and Deuteronomy), that dictate kosher (literally, "acceptable") food preparation. To the orthodox, observing these food preparation mandates is more than mere sound public health policy—they are a call to be faithful to the holiness of the Torah. Food in this case is not just nutrition, but worship.

There are seven major fasting days in Judaism, lasting usually from sunset to sunrise, except for Yom Kippur, which is traditionally 25 hours long. Fasting in Judaism is often associated with grieving and loss (reflective of David's fasting over the loss of Saul; 2 Samuel 1:12). There are many important psycho–emotional subtleties to Jewish fasting. Food is also found in Jewish myth as a means of celebration, remembrance, reflection, and mourning.

Let us keep in mind one of the admonitions that the Jewish prophets (the meshiachs) directed at the Jewish elite: their obsession with animal sacrifice. Besides feeling that the Jewish rulers had essentially abandoned social welfare for the needy and afflicted, the Prophets Hosea, Micah, and Isaiah rebuked the leaders for their mass slaughtering practices; they felt the rulers had become too ritual–obsessed while no longer serving the common person with the true religious offerings of hope, charity, and love.

Some of the early Christians appropriated the Laws of Kashrut for themselves and in subsequent formalizations by the Roman Catholic Church. These laws ultimately became the Western Catholic observances of abstention and lent. Just like Jewish dietary laws, Christian fasting distinguished the religiously faithful from the disloyal and the earnest from the disingenuous.

Food is presented in some remarkable ways in the Christian books. Five loaves and two fishes feed "five thousand men . . . to say nothing of women and children" (Matthew 14:21).[2] How the fish were cooked is curiously omitted from Matthew's work, as over five thousand people eating raw fish would have certainly been an unheard of event in ancient Palestine.

Jesus also counsels the disciples earlier in this Gospel not to be too concerned with storing provisions: "That is why I am telling you not to worry about your life and what you are to eat, nor about your body and what you are to wear. Surely life is more than food, and the body more than clothing!" (Matthew 6:25). This may be one of Matthew's ways of portraying Jesus as a Jewish reformer, defying the emphasis of Kosher Law.

The climax of food as metaphor occurs in Matthew when Jesus and the twelve dine together at Passover. The Eucharist gets instituted from the story found in Matthew 26:26 as the bread becomes Jesus' body and the wine his blood. This metaphoric use of food by Matthew is a stark statement reinforcing Matthew's rhetorical objective: Jesus has become the new food for the Israelites. As Passover commemorates Moses freeing his people, the Eucharist signifies the new Moses (Jesus) liberating his people to a new age of spiritual understanding. Matthew is certainly not known for his subtlety in making the controversial point that Judaism is forever changed through Jesus' legacy, one that has gained Matthew considerable attention as anti-Jewish.

The controversy over observing a kosher food tradition was a central problem in the early formation of Christianity. The Palestinian Jews, who included Peter, John, and James (Jesus' brother), were all faithful to the Laws of Moses in the Torah. For Paul (Saul) of Tarsus, Jewish missionary to the Gentiles, having to force the Goyim to observe all the strict rules of the Jews was contrary to keeping them as adherents to this developing branch of neo-Judaism (now called Christianity). Paul insists on his faithfulness to Torah, holding himself up as a paragon of pharisaic dutifulness. For Paul, the Jews were to continue observing the Laws of Torah, but for the pagans the rules would have to be modified.

In Acts we read that a compromise is reached in the first Christian council in Jerusalem. The new recommendations that Paul will present to the gentiles regarding food are not to eat any blood or meat from strangled animals and not to receive meat that has been sacrificed to foreign idols (Acts 15:19). Paul knew that if the rules were too strict, especially in relation to food, he would never be able to keep the diverse congregations together.

In Islam, the Muslim faithful also are influenced by the Jewish kosher recommendations. Called *halaal* in Arabic, it is the same concept of allowable foods for the faithful; that which is *haraam* is not allowable. The Muslims would eventually modify the laws of Kashrut slightly and allow shellfish and seafood, for example. In Islam, just as in Judaism, observing food restrictions and fasting is an important part of religious loyalty. For many Muslims the apex of this observance occurs during the holy month of Ramadan.

Certainly in the monotheistic creeds, food is central to the faithfulness of the religiously observant. This has been altered with time since spiritual tenets have taken a backseat to social concerns, and the original spiritual function of some religious sects has been abducted by unbridled commercialism and the bane of theological literalism, at least in post–industrial communities.

The focus on food and religious observance is replicated, albeit for somewhat diverse reasons, with the Eastern disciplines of Hinduism and Buddhism. Although there are important distinctions one can make between the religious observances of these two creeds, they are in consort on their food laws enough to make some basic generalizations:

1. The beginning precept in both religious schools is the concept of ahimsa, non–harming. This is a central core attitude towards all life, one of non–violence, non–malice. Since it requires a certain violent act to take an animal's life, it is forbidden in the essential teachings of these schools.
2. Animals are considered sentient beings and, as such, contain consciousness. To kill anything with consciousness is to promote bad karma for yourself and interfere with the evolutionary trajectory of the ever–evolving life form.
3. Eating animals promotes animal behaviors in humans. There is a certain vibration to meat that is corrupting to orthodox Buddhist and Hindu students.
4. Taking intoxicants (alcohol, drugs) and eating meat and heat–producing foods such as garlic and onions, stir up animal passions and precipitate karmic–producing actions and are to be avoided. This is especially mandated for monastics who are devoted to dispassion and transcendence. The idea is that what you take in

affects your consciousness, and the idea behind most of the Eastern religions is a purification of consciousness.

Many Buddhists believe that the Shakyamuni Buddha lived as animals prior to his various human incarnations and that keeping to vegetarianism therefore honors his legacy. There are some Buddhists (and others) who believe that one of the root causes of so much world violence is the pervasive violence towards animals. With this ethos, living as a vegetarian helps to promote world peace.

Although most Buddhist monastics are committed to vegetarianism, in traditional sects monastics are expected to beg for their monetary and nutritional necessities. Since they are to thankfully accept anyone's contribution, they may receive meat as an offering from the public. As an expression of gratitude, they would be encouraged by their teachers to eat it, most likely with substantial prayer accompanying the meal.

In Hinduism, ayurveda, which is the traditional health system of India, is a philosophy largely devoted to food recommendations. Depending upon your individual element type, called your dosha, and the season of the year, you decide which food choices and combinations will be the most healthful, often with the assistance of an ayurvedic doctor. Meats usually are taken only moderately unless one is undergoing a systemic cleansing where vegetarianism is mandated. Many swamis, who usually are vegetarian, prefer meatless dishes but do take dairy, as they consider it to be good for the energetic (pranic) essence of the body.

Just like Buddhists, many devout Hindus are predominantly vegetarian. This was not so in the early days of Hinduism, when the religion was dominated by the Brahmin caste. In the sixth century B.C.E., Buddhism and Jainism were the dominant religious forces in India and South Central Asia. It was from their influence that Hinduism got much of its contemporary focus on ethics and devotion to the Divine. With that said, I recall the words a dear swami told me years ago: "If we [swamis] can't change the vibration of a little piece of meat now and then with our prayers of gratitude and love, we should just hang it up and join the circus." True liberation is not being a total captive to either vegetarianism or carnivorous eating.

Food is utilized in many traditions throughout the world as a religious observance. The use of fasting for devotional means is common and has been shown to have significant health benefits, as well.

It is important to keep in mind that fasting should not be approached merely as a one-dimensional activity; fasting from certain foods should accompany fasting from certain thoughts, such as worry, anxiety, fear, enmity, and rancor. The following section will assist you in customizing fasts to your needs. Remember to be patient and gradually introduce your dietary changes. Fasting should be for a purpose and for a predetermined length of time. As always, if you need assistance in fasting because of health concerns, confer with a trusted healthcare advisor. Remember: things that progress gradually last longer, so be patient.

10

The Seven Types of Fasts

ONE SHOULD PREPARE THE BODY PRIOR TO FASTING. FOR FIVE TO seven days prior to embarking upon any fast, eliminate refined sugar, fast foods, and fried foods (interesting how these three things are often found together). It is suggested that a person embarking on a fast increase his daily intake of purified water and, if possible, cease taking any caffeinated beverages. Although many people who consume refined sugar and caffeine daily will find the first two to three days difficult, it is worth persevering as the eventual results are well worth it.

Keep in mind that it is not recommended that one go completely without nutrients, which is a very specialized and highly disciplined fast, requiring ample preparation and guidance, and certainly not recommended for anyone with a serious medical condition. The closest we will get in our seven fasts is with #1, the Pure Fast. The other six fasts are, in effect, preparations for the Pure Fast and perfectly viable in and of themselves; not everyone flourishes on the Pure Fast. As always, pay attention to your specific needs.

People often comment in amazement, "I was shocked at how much energy I had!" when they complete their first fast. Therefore, the first issue to clarify is that smart fasting does not make one weak.[1] Simplifying the diet and enjoying fresh, healthy foods is like natural medicine for the body's cells. It is also very sensible to eat according to one's metabolic type during the fast, emphasizing the nutrients that work best with a specific metabolic constitution.

Building vs. Purifying

Fasts that contain whole grains, legumes, dairy, and meat broths are essentially building fasts (anabolic)—for the purpose of strengthening and repairing tissues such as muscle, fascia, bone, ligament, and tendon. Fasts that contain vegetables, vegetable juices, green foods, fruits, and most mushrooms are essentially cleansing fasts (catabolic)—for the purpose of purification and reduction. Many of the fasts listed here are a sensible combination of the two, as both processes are interactively taking place in the body all the time and because many people are a mixture, to some degree, of protein–dominant and carbohydrate–dominant types.

Here are some fundamental ideas to consider when engaged in a fast:

1. Keep your mind on the Source behind your health; there is a life force that is sustaining you above and beyond nutrients. A fast should help you get in touch with that sacred energy; your daily spiritual practice helps you *stay* in touch with it. If you don't have a spiritual practice that works for you, now would be the time to find one.

2. Moderate your activities, especially the longer the fast and the newer you are to it. For the following seven fasts, the lower the number of the fast, the more relaxed you should make your activities; no heavy exertion or labor, and only leisurely, enjoyable exercise. For example, The Whole Grains Helper (#6) is more apt to sustain generous physical activity than is The Phytolic Filtrator (#2) for the novice. Once your body gets acclimated to better nutrition, which yields more efficient digestion and less metabolic by-products, you should get ample energy from the lower numbered fasts.

3. For fasts numbered 3–5, a colonic irrigation treatment is *highly* recommended. A well-trained and experienced practitioner of colon hydrotherapy or natural–medicine clinician may have further advice for your specific needs. Make sure that you do not become reliant upon colonic irrigations—they are meant only to jump-start peristalsis, your body's natural muscular movement

of the gastrointestinal tract. Do not use them as a persistent surrogate for normal, regular bowel evacuations.

4. It is better to eat small amounts more frequently than to overload the system at any given meal. A general rule–of–thumb for estimating an appropriate serving size is this.[2]

    - Keep portions of protein to about the size of your open palm, from wrist crease to creases of your first knuckles.
    - Keep cereals and grains to as much as two cupped hands can hold as a maximum single serving. Remember to ask yourself, "Do I want to use my maximum with one nutrient?"
    - Servings of fruits or vegetables should approximate the size of your whole fist or a bit bigger.
    - Oil, butter, ghee, and dressings should correspond to the size of your thumb. For oils and dressings: from the knuckle crease at your palm to the tip; for butter and ghee: the size of your thumb from the tip to the second (distal) knuckle crease.
    - Sauces should cover the area no bigger than your four fingers touching, from the edge of the palm to the tip of the pinky.
    - Sweets should not exceed the size of your pinky finger's length and circumference.
    - When you are engaged in a fast and unable to escape to the top of the mountain by yourself (meaning you still have job and family obligations), take food with you. Eat small amounts on a frequent basis until your body adjusts. Taking smaller portions of the best quality nutrients is one of the keys to gaining better health.

5. If you must take a caffeinated beverage, green tea is ideal (maximum: 2–3 cups daily). Second is black unsweetened organic coffee (1 cup, approximately 8–10 ounces), with black tea (1 cup) as the third alternative. One way to decrease the potential acidity of black tea, which many are sensitive to, is to mix ½ black tea with ½ herbal tea. Another preference is to add both fresh–squeezed lemon and lime juice. Experiment and find your own affinity.

6. Drink plenty of purified water—*at least* 1.5 liters a day (about 6 cups), with 3 liters being ideal in hotter seasons and climates.

Water with fresh lemon or lime is a good systemic cleanser.

7. Always allow time in-between fasts. The quick rule of thumb is this: twice as many off (the fast) as on. If you fast for 4 days, leave *at least* 8 days recovery time before you start your next one. When you are on the first day of breaking your fast, take predigested dairy of a skim milk variety (yogurt, cottage cheese), or 1/2 teaspoon of ghee in a standard pot of tea; introduce heavier foods after 2–3 days and very moderately. Continue to drink an abundance of purified water and maintain lemon or lime water 2–4 days after your fast. Remember: take citrus and dairy at opposite ends of the day (or at least at different meal times) and never together.

The Seven Fasts

#7: The Whole Grains and Produce Booster

This is often the easiest starting place for most people. For three days prior to this fast you should cut out all alcohol and refined sugar from your diet (that means you have to read labels as to what is in your food)[5] and keep it that way throughout the duration of the fast.

Low level: for *three* days eat nothing but cooked whole grains and fresh produce. The produce should be a mixture of cooked (preferably steamed) and raw. You can add a little ghee (clarified butter) and spices as needed. From waking in the morning until three hours before bedtime, you can take small amounts (4–6 ounces) of plain organic yogurt, eaten by itself as a snack. Do not eat anything three hours prior to sleeping; herbal teas are acceptable. If you are a protein-dominant type, you may need to eat small amounts of nut butter or a low-fat cheese at each meal.

Medium Level: For *five* days eat nothing but cooked whole grains and fresh produce. You can add ghee (clarified butter) and spices as needed. Yogurt is acceptable during the first two days only.

High Level: For *seven* days eat nothing but cooked whole grains and fresh produce. Do not take yogurt during this level of fast.

#6: The Whole Grain Domain

Low level: For *three* days eat nothing but cooked whole grains. This includes breads of sprouted grain and grain combinations, such as quinoa and millet, brown rice and spelt, oats and amaranth, and others. You may add various spices to taste: ginger, cumin, tumeric, cinnamon, cardamom, nutmeg, mace, sea salt, pepper, and so on. You can add organic ghee, olive oil, or sesame oil in small amounts, as desired.

Medium Level: For *five* days eat nothing but cooked whole grains (no breads). Follow above recommendations: olive oil or sesame oil for the first two days only. Ghee is allowable in very small amounts.

High Level: For *seven* days eat nothing but cooked whole grains (no breads). Ghee is permissible during the first three days. Add spices as desired.

Note: if you are a protein-dominant metabolic type, you may want to add small amounts of dairy during the first few days and gradually wean yourself off as you go. Pay attention to the signals your body sends during the fast.

#5: The Produce Purge

Ewwww . . . scary word "purge," eh? For some it is, but don't let that deter you. This is a very revitalizing fast, introducing a good amount of healthful phytochemicals (plant chemicals) into the system. This is a great way to get more soluble and insoluble fiber through the gastrointestinal tract, acting as a kind of natural roto-rooter for your internal plumbing. Also, your cells will be happy with these plant nutrients.

Low Level: For *three* days, eat nothing but vegetables: raw, steamed, and stir-fried (ghee, olive, or sesame oils are preferable), and fresh fruits. The first day can include small amounts of whole grains for first-timers and mixed metabolic types. Fruits are best in the morning and last thing in the evening (except melon, which for most is usually best in the morning only).

Medium Level: For *five* days, eat vegetables: raw or steamed (not stir-fried). Take fruits in the morning or throughout the day, at least ninety minutes after vegetables. Small amounts of ghee and olive oil are fine for the first two days. Season your food to taste.

High Level: For seven days eat nothing but raw (50%) and steamed (50%) vegetables. Only protein-dominants may use oils; spices are okay, including small amounts of low-sodium soy sauce and tamari. Eat fruit in small amounts throughout the day and drink an abundance of water. If your body has been sluggish or prone to constipation prior to this fast, you may need to take a colonic on the first and third or fourth day, depending on how you feel.

#4: The Citrus Simplifier

Low Level: for three days eat only citrus fruits: grapefruit, oranges, and tangerines. Because of the high citric acid content of lemons and limes, it is recommended that you juice them with grapefruit and orange or mix them with water. Take herbal teas, if you like. Each evening prior to bedtime, take 1 teaspoon of olive oil. You will feel hungrier sooner on this fast, so keep citrus fruit close by and enjoy as much as you need.

Medium Level: for five days eat only citrus fruits, especially oranges and tangerines. For the first two evenings, take 2 teaspoons of olive oil, then 1 teaspoon for two evenings, and nothing for the last evening. Drink plenty of water and herbal tea.

High Level: for seven days eat citrus fruits, especially oranges and tangerines. Take 1 teaspoon of olive oil at bedtime for the first three days, no oils on days 4, 5, 6; 3 teaspoons of olive oil on the last night before bedtime. Drink lots of water each day.

#3: The Apple Diet Riot

This is a very cleansing diet. Ensure that the apples are organic and eat the peelings. Red apples are recommended as the bulwark of the diet, but a few fujis or green varieties thrown in here and there, I have found, break up the monotony of this challenging fast. There are only two levels to this fast.

Medium Level: Eat apples—lots of them—for three days. Take 1 tablespoon of olive oil at bedtime for the first two nights; for the last night, take 3 tablespoons of olive oil. Make sure that you get a colonic on the second day; you could feel very unwell on the third day if you do not, as lots of toxins could be moving through your system. Drink plenty of water and herbal tea.

High Level: You should not attempt this fast without a few successful completions of the three-day version. For five days, eat nothing but apples. Take 1 tablespoon of olive oil every evening for the first three evenings; on the fourth evening take 2 tablespoons; on the fifth evening take 3 tablespoons. Drink lots of water and herbal tea. If you need a protein snack during this fast, eat raw almonds or pistachio nuts soaked overnight in sea salt water, or roasted organic soybeans.

#2: The Phytolic Filtrator

Low Level: For *three* days eat only green foods, including steamed dark leafy-greens, micro-algae, celery, asparagus, artichokes, Brussels sprouts, sprouts (alfalfa, clover, and so forth), romaine lettuce, and the like. For fruits: green grapes, green apples, kiwi, and green tomatoes (vine-ripened only). Green food supplements in the form of wheat grass juice, spirulina, chlorella, and wild blue-green algae can be taken in the morning or early afternoon. The addition of mushrooms (raw, steamed, or boiled) is acceptable anytime and, if needed, small amounts of olive oil.

Medium Level: for *five* days eat only green foods, with the same guidance as the previous level. If protein is needed, take raw almonds or pistachio nuts soaked overnight in salt water, and/or miso soup.

High Level: for *seven* days eat only green foods, with the same guidance as the previous level. Make sure to take a colonic irrigation by the end of the fourth day. Drink lots of water and herbal tea; keep your mind focused on the Divine.

#1: The Pure Fast

Low Level: Make sure you have successfully completed any three of
the previous six fasts prior to attempting this one. For *three* days take
nothing but fruit and vegetable juices,[4] herbal teas, green food micro-
algae, and wheat grass juice.

Medium Level: For *five* days take nothing but fruit and vegetable
juices,[5] herbal teas, micro-algae, and wheat grass juice. If you need a
protein, take miso soup and/or the broth of free-range chickens or wild
(not farmed) fish.

High Level: For *seven* days take nothing but fruit and vegetable juices,[6]
herbal teas, green food micro-algae, and wheat grass juice. If you need
a protein, take miso soup.

You have many choices at your disposal. The crucial point is to get
busy trying these ideas out and making them your own. All of the ideas
presented throughout the chapters are suggestions and not meant to be
inflexible rules, although the repetitive recommendations are the closest we will get to nutritional dogma. You should implement a variety of
approaches to see what works best for your specific situation.

11

A History of Food Narrative

SOMEWHERE AROUND 12,000 YEARS AGO HUMANS DEVELOPED A WAY to domesticate wild plants, creating the base for agriculture. This was a significant expansion of human control over environment. Prior to this, as the standard archaeological myth goes, humans relied on foraging and were at the mercy of their environment for the survival of our species. Taking control of the production of food and animals transformed the prehistoric societies from being nomadic to being sedentary, which ultimately sets the stage for cities, buildings, temples, governments, and all the places we associate with communal activity today—Chuck E. Cheese, K–mart, The Piggly Wiggly, Bloomingdale's, to name a few.

How this process took place is easier to determine than why. There are about eight scientifically acceptable hypotheses that explain why we became a farming people.[1] Scientists think that there was a diffusion of knowledge, simultaneously developing throughout populated regions, passing from one group to another the knowledge of how to control plant growth. Another explanation, although not accepted in the mainstream, is that there were much older, sophisticated cultures with established agricultural and horticultural practices already in place, and this information was passed from generation to generation through farmers and teachers in both oral and written forms. The latter theory accounts for the lost civilizations of Lemuria, Mu, Atlantis, etc.

One of the oldest areas of crop domestication that the archaeological record reveals is in the Levant.[2] This is the place that many in the archaeological community refer to as the cradle of modern civilization. Uncovered in this broad region are some of the oldest organized communities known to date. Even though the standard viewpoint is that all life emanated from Africa, when we were in our grunting and wobbly bipedal pre–hominid phase, the cultural evolution of modern man is given its roots in the Levant (stay tuned . . . subject to further revision).

The first domesticated crops appear to be wild cereal and legume harvests. Various combinations of wild wheat, barley, oats, lentils, chick peas, and field peas have been discovered in numerous excavation sites. These, by the way, are carbohydrates—our oldest domesticated plant-food sources.

Prior to this, we were likely eating whatever we could catch or collect—animals, insects, herbs, and fruits. Yes, much of what passes today as ghastly reality-TV entertainment—the eating of worms, spiders, bugs, and anything else that looks like it just crawled out of Indiana Jones' footlocker—is edible and has been in our food chain for thousands of years. The next time you see a creepy–crawly don't think DEET, think "bon appetite."

But back to our story. Each area of the developing world that had significant populations also had a grain staple or two. Even today in China, one of the characters representing food is the same one that represents grain.

Historically, in East Asia the grain staple was rice; in Southwest Asia it was wheat; in Africa it was sorghum and varieties of millet; in the Americas it was maize (corn). The crops of Southwest Asia influenced the agriculture of Europe, and we find wheat and barley as some of the earliest phytocentric nutrients for this region. Later, the cereal spelt was cultivated and became a significant food source in the middle ages of central Europe.

No matter where we investigate—Egypt, China, South America, the Middle East—all of the ancient societies appear to have eaten whole-grain carbohydrates, with very few exceptions. Keep in mind that we are talking about whole grains, not the refined variety so widespread today. The refining process comes much later, along with sugar cane, and with it a multitude of health problems.

Meats have also been standard dietary fare for most cultures. Traditionally, there have been very few truly vegan societies, except in times of dire straits or special circumstances. There have been a few cultural subdivisions that have shunned animal foods for religious reasons, but they have not been reflective of the community at large. The majority of these cultural subdivisions have included dairy products to some degree, eliminating them from being truly vegan.

Some people like to idealize aboriginal cultures, be they of the Americas, Australia, or Asia, as wholly vegetarian. The truth is they used to, and still do, eat various animals while retaining a very robust shamanistic religious tradition. We could include the ancient Israelites (meats, with numerous dietary restrictions), the early Christians (both Palestinian and gentile), the Sufis, and the assorted mystics from Afghanistan to Egypt in this list of meat-eating religious groups. As mentioned, there have been exceptions to this; some spiritual sects chose vegetarianism as the ideal dietary standard within all the mentioned traditions.

This was before the mass commercialization of domesticated animals, prior to the chemical revolution, when there was still a wild, organic element to the meat—when hunters would take the animals prayerfully, as an offering from the Creator to the community. Huge agribusiness operations have built up since the industrial revolution with thousands of animals in one location. As a consequence, the addition of growth hormones, antibiotics, and other chemical agents has made much of the standard meat supply problematic. Witness the recent episodes of Mad Cow Disease; here the bovine immune system is reacting against being fed ground-up parts of other animals—in many cases, other cows. We cannot disregard the herbivore's digestive biology in this way. There have also been problems with poultry and pork provisions in some areas.

This mass conglomeration of animals in one space is not reflective of nature's way. It is not too often that you will encounter 3,500 chickens in one enclosed space in nature. When one bird gets sick, the pathogen quickly spreads to other birds who are confined in commercial cages. This happens with all animals (including us humans) and makes for potential difficulties in mass meat production. This is not even consid-

ering the occasional unsanitary meat processing and packing component, which is frequently exposed in acclaimed books and news ar-
ticles. The moral of this story: choose your meat sources very carefully.

In the 1950s and prior, most chickens were raised for their eggs. After
the invention of the pressure cooker, a certain Southern "colonel" found
out that he could fry chicken quickly, and with the addition of his "11
secret herbs," a big bird biz was born. Fried chicken flesh is now hugely
popular in overseas countries (China is one of the most burgeoning
markets), as are other fast-food businesses. These are some of the same
countries that once were paragons of good health and now are showing
signs of some of the same health problems that fast-food-loving Americans exhibit.

Americans love meat. Our national adage might be "If a little is good,
a lot must be really good, and all-you-can-eat is the best!" Compared to
other countries, we just may be overdoing it in our perpetual fascina-
tion with 20-ounce steaks and 25-piece chicken dinners. According to
the USDA,

> "Now more than ever, America is a nation of meat eaters. In
> 2000, total meat consumption (red meat, poultry, and fish)
> reached 195 pounds (boneless, trimmed-weight equiva-
> lent) per person, 57 pounds above average annual con-
> sumption in the 1950s. Each American consumed an
> average of 7 pounds more red meat than in the 1950s, 46
> pounds more poultry, and 4 pounds more fish and shell-
> fish. Rising consumer incomes, especially with the increase
> in two-income households, and meat prices in the 1990s
> that were often at 50-year lows, when adjusted for inflation,
> explain much of the increase in meat consumption. In
> addition, the meat industry has provided scores of new
> brand-name, value-added products processed for consum-
> ers' convenience, as well as a host of products for foodservice
> operators."[3]

Perhaps we can thank a certain "colonel" for our 46-pound-per-person increase of poultry consumption, but nobody is forcing us to chomp an extra pound of chicken legs or stuff our gullet with 20 ounces of bloody sirloin. Have you heard about the obesity epidemic and soaring rates of hypertension and high blood pressure? But surely that is not going to dissuade a person from that extra thigh, is it? The problem unquestionably is excess consumption of poor quality foods.

In order to understand how we got into this predicament, it would be helpful to look at a food timeline. Our abbreviated food timeline picks up in earnest at the commencement of the industrial revolution in England. Josiah Wedgewood and his companions, the Staffordshire potters, employed the use of waterwheels and windmills to turn and blend their pottery materials in England, early 1700's. The British were learning much about pottery by carefully examining the craftwork they received from chinaware caches of the East India Trading Company. Their craftsmanship became so refined that when machinery was developed, they could easily transfer their handiwork into mass production. After 1850, mechanical assistance in ceramics manufacturing became common, and the availability of inexpensive crockery made eating and drinking much more sanitary.

From 1750 to about 1900, farmers would increase crop production dramatically. By employing a crop rotating system that utilizes a four-year cycle—turnips or another root crop the first year, barley the second, clover or grass the third, and wheat in the fourth, farmers no longer had to let the land go fallow. This meant that production could escalate and so could profits. The demand for food increased as cities became more populated with industrial workers. Machinery was invented to assist farmers with their ever-growing troubles of feeding more people.

One of the most important inventions was the advent of commercial refrigeration. This development arose from the spreading of commercial ice plants. As the water supplies became more polluted because of industrial expansion, the ice business became infused with problems. The next logical step was to mechanically manufacture ice, paving the way for mechanical refrigeration. The first industry to recognize the implications of refrigeration was the breweries. Starting in New York in 1870 and expanding to the northeastern states, refrigeration changed the nature of American brewing. It was not until the turn of the twentieth century that the meat–packing industry adopted refrigeration, with Chicago's immense meat markets leading the way.

The invention of refrigeration technologies applied to trains created a wider distribution of food products across the country. Starting with milk and butter products in the 1840s, perishable meats were added about twenty years later, and by the 1870s, meats and other perishable goods were slowly opening up markets across the country.

The invention of the home refrigerator was probably one of the most monumental developments to expand agricultural markets and affect family health habits. In 1921 there were approximately 5,000 mechanical refrigerators, but that number would grow dramatically in ten years to one million. Around 1937–1938 there were an estimated six million refrigerator units sold in the U.S. This meant fewer trips to the local market and more available pre–packaged foods on hand for the consumer.

At the turn of the twentieth century, we have the beginnings of some of today's dilemmas: family farms deteriorating with less urban land going toward food production and the escalating competition from expanding agribusiness behemoths.

Corporations rely on complex strategies, many of which have parallels with the military culture. One military strategy that has proven effective for millennia is to control the opponent's food and water supplies. "Take them by their stomach," the martial edict goes, "and their will soon follows." As we traded agricultural customs for technological ones, at the expense of some common–sense traditions, we headed down a murky road of disorder. It would take some time for this to be apparent, as well as the end of a world war symbolizing just how far we have pushed technology to the top of our psychosocial hierarchy.

After the explosions on Hiroshima and Nagasaki, technology heralded itself as the bold new deity of the twentieth century. This was a fierce, wrathful Old Testament god with no patience for graven images and a people who did not obey its every command. Even today with the humanoid voices emanating from computers worldwide, there is still a strange familiarity to the pseudo–humanity of it all. Recall this exchange from *2001: A Space Odyssey*: (For those who have not read the book or seen the movie, HAL is a computer.)

Dave Bowman: Hello, HAL do you read me, HAL?
HAL: Affirmative, Dave, I read you.

Dave Bowman: Open the pod bay doors, HAL.
HAL: I'm sorry Dave, I'm afraid I can't do that.

Dave Bowman: What's the problem?
HAL: I think you know what the problem is just as well as I do.

Dave Bowman: What are you talking about, HAL?
HAL: This mission is too important for me to allow you to jeopardize it.

Dave Bowman: I don't know what you're talking about, HAL.
HAL: I know you and Frank were planning to disconnect me, and I'm afraid that's something I cannot allow to happen.

Dave Bowman: Where the hell'd you get that idea, HAL?
HAL: Dave, although you took thorough precautions in the pod against my hearing you, I could see your lips move.[4]

Although technology has brought many comforts and conveniences, it has also carried considerable problems. It is a given that nothing is perfect in the world of human invention; however, when it comes to things that directly affect our health and well-being, most of us would prefer the imperfections to be on the more conservative side.

After WWII the chemical industries flourished, both in medicine and in agriculture. Without combat as the grounds for chemical production, the big question remained: What would the expanding poison-making businesses manufacture without an enemy to target? The answer would spawn three giant industries: agricultural poisons, pharmaceuticals, and food additives.

Technology kept up with the demand as well as the inventiveness of entrepreneurs' savoir-faire, modifying food supplies and creating markets. With the increased use of tractors and self-propelled combines on the farm, the problem that arose was one of excess—we were producing a surplus of food. This, integrated with the new chemicalization of agriculture with DDT, anhydrous ammonia (nitrogen fertilizer), and fungicides, made for abundance in the fields.

Just as the livestock and poultry industries expanded and became bigger operations to leverage their competitive edge, the agriculture enterprises also expanded, with the Goliaths eventually terminating the Davids. Today, in order to compete in the market, most full-time farms need to be 2,500 acres or bigger. This has reduced the competition significantly.

Today, the developments in food technologies are changing monthly. There are an unprecedented number of chemicals in food and beverage supplies, as well as numerous governmental agencies appointed to research and regulate safety. Just a brief survey of the bureaucratic tentacles reveals a database of acronyms: FDA, DHHS, USDA, FSIS, EPA, APHIS, CDC, NIH, CSREES, AMS, ERS, GIPSA, NMFS, FFDCA, FMIA, and the list goes on.

The expanding technologic area affecting food supplies is the science of genetic modification. The exploration of genetically modified organisms (GMOs) in the food sciences is a controversial topic for the twenty-first century, prompting the question, "Just how much can science mutate the DNA of foods without creating a health-hazard?" A new documentary entitled "The Future of Food" explores the difficulties inherent in the new science of genetic modification.

GMO foods have been legally introduced to commercial food supplies since 1997. Although there are currently no federal governmental mandates for disclosing GMO contents in products, states like Vermont and California have passed legislation requiring labeling of GMO foods within their borders. The health risks of GMO foods are still unclear.

With the escalation in scientific developments, food supplies have become increasingly altered from their natural state. Much of what was once organically grown in the backyard is now artificially cultivated in laboratories. Animals are often suffering an abnormal upbringing, many without the space needed for adequate exercise or the foods that fit their inherent dietary preferences. The proliferation of using chemicals in raising livestock, as well as aberrant feeding practices, has yet to see its full impact.

The most pressing requirement for America's stewardship of its natural resources is a greater awareness of its unbridled consumerism. We must respect the land and the animals, just as our tribal ancestors did, not expecting science to save us from the troubles born of abandoning common sense. To paraphrase the wisdom of a tribal elder, "It is only when the white man has no clean air to breathe, no good water to drink, and no food that is edible that he will realize you cannot breathe, drink, or eat his precious money."

In this new era, we must realize that financial considerations have to take a back seat to ethical ones. We must come back to the wisdom of nature, learning how to maintain harmony with a system that is pre-existent to humankind. We must learn from our past errors of arrogance and technocentric hubris, realizing that technology can only go so far in fixing the problems that misuse of same multiplies. May the twenty-first century clarify for humans that nature is the best teacher and that all our inventions should compliment the natural way of things. We must encourage the new generation of scientists to be students of nature's intelligence—not mere manipulators or educated scavengers.

Science has done many wonderful things to advance our knowledge of the physical world when implemented by people with respectful and honorable intentions. We must encourage more of the same while disallowing the old destructive archetype to flourish. Whether it is food for our bodies, minds, or spirits, we are now called to culturally mature and find a Source existing behind all life, which—if understood properly and revered wisely—will change the world as we know it.

12

A History of Food Timeline[1]

7500 B.C.E.

Chili pepper, whose active ingredient is capsicum, "has been known since the beginning of civilization in the Western Hemisphere. It has been a part of the human diet since about 7500 B.C. (MacNeish 1964). Ancient ancestors of the native peoples took the wild chile piquin and selected for the many various types known today. Heiser (1976) states that apparently between 5200 and 3400 B.C., the Native Americans were growing chile plants.[2]

6000 B.C.E.

Lima Beans are being cultivated in Peru.

4000 B.C.E.

Dates are being cultivated around the Persian Gulf and are revered as a symbol of fertility.

4000 B.C.E.

Citrus fruits are cultivated in the areas of Mesopotamia. "The citron's place of origin is unknown, but seeds were found in Mesopotamian excavations dating back to 4000 B.C. The armies of Alexander the Great are thought to have carried the citron to the Mediterranean region about 300 B.C. A Jewish coin struck in 136 B.C. bore a representation of the citron on one side. A Chinese writer in A.D. 300 spoke of a gift of "40 Chinese bushels of citrons from Ta–ch'in" in A.D. 284. Ta–ch'in is understood to mean the Roman Empire. The citron was a staple commercial food item in Rome in A.D. 301."[3]

3500 B.C.E.

Cultivation of the **olive** tree in the Mediterranean. "Some historians . . . claim that archaeological discoveries prove that wild olive trees existed before civilization in Crete and that their cultivation began during the Paleolithic and Neolithic periods, i.e., between 3500 and 5000 B.C. From Crete the trees spread to Egypt (2000 B.C.), and thereafter to the islands, Asia Minor, Palestine, and mainland Greece (1800 B.C.)."[4]

3000 B.C.E.

Wild garlic begins to be cultivated and dispersed. "Garlic is among the oldest known horticultural crops. In the Old World, Egyptian and Indian cultures referred to garlic 5,000 years ago, and there is clear historical evidence for its use by the Babylonians 4,500 years ago and by the Chinese 2,000 years ago. Some writings suggest that garlic was grown in China as far back as 4,000 years ago. Today, garlic grows wild only in Central Asia (centered in Kyrgyzstan, Tajikistan, Turkmenistan, and Uzbekistan). Earlier in history garlic grew wild over a much larger region. In fact, wild garlic may have occurred in an area from China to India to Egypt to the Ukraine."[5]

2900 B.C.E.

The edible **fig** proliferates throughout the Middle East and eventually the Mediterranean: "The common fig probably originated in the fertile part of southern Arabia (Solms–Laubach 1885). Ancient records indicate both King Urukagina of the Sumarian era (2900 B.C.) and the Assyrians (2000 B.C.) were familiar with it. No records exist of its introduction to this area, but the caprifig, ancestor of the edible fig, is still found there growing wild. From southern Arabia, the Bahra tribe brought the fig to ancient Idumaea and Oelsyria (Lagarde 1881). Over a period of several centuries, it slowly spread from there to Syria and the Mediterranean coast. Once figs reached the coast, they rapidly spread throughout the Mediterranean region aided by the maritime nations. They were known in Crete by 1600 B.C."[6]

2700 B.C.E.

There is **wine** in the Nile Delta in Egypt. The grapes, which were likely transported from the areas in and around Israel and Jordan, would take centuries to be cultivated by Egyptian farmers.

2000 B.C.E.

Technology to produce **butter** from domesticated animals is developed: "The earliest details of [butter manufacturing] are derived from the Arabs and Syrians, who appear to be as well satisfied with the original process of making butter as they are with other habits, since they have remained unchanged for centuries. The original practice of the Arabs and Syrians, so far as is known, was to use a vessel made from goatskin for a churn. The animal was skinned and the skin sewed up tight, leaving an opening only at the left foreleg, where the cream was poured in. The 'churn' was then suspended from the tent poles and swung until the 'butter comes.' This, incidentally, is the earliest known process of making butter."[7] This is not far removed from the process used today in many developing countries.

2000 B.C.E.

The pods of the **carob** tree (*Ceratonia siliqua*) are utilized for carbohydrate energy: "Carob is native to the eastern Mediterranean, probably the Middle East, where it has been in cultivation for at least 4,000 years. The plant was well known to the ancient Greeks, who planted seeds of this plant in Greece and Italy. There are references to carob in the Bible. For example, this plant is also called St. John's bread or locust bean because the pods were once thought to have been the locusts that were eaten by John the Baptist in the wilderness. Carob seeds were used to weight gold, hence the word *carat*. Mohammed's army ate *kharoub*, and Arabs planted the crop in northern Africa and Spain (Moors), along with citrus (*Citrus*) and olives (*Olea*). Spaniards carried carob to Mexico and South America, and the British took carob to South Africa, India, and Australia."[8]

1500 B.C.E.

Horseradish is used in both culinary and medicinal applications: "The Egyptians knew about horseradish as far back as 1500 B.C.E. Early Greeks used it as a rub for low-back pain and as an aphrodisiac. Jews still use it during Passover Seders as one of the bitter herbs. Some Greeks used horseradish syrup as an expectorant cough medicine; others were convinced it cured everything from rheumatism to tuberculosis. Legend has it the Delphic oracle told Apollo, *The radish is worth its weight in lead, the beet its weight in silver, the horseradish its weight in gold.*"[9]

Circa ninth century

Sausage is mentioned in Homer's *Odyssey*. Smoked and cured meats are a part of many cultural traditions throughout the World.

700 B.C.E.

Cinnamon is treasured for its flavor and medicinal benefits: "The Egyptians used cinnamon and cassia along with myrrh in embalming, perhaps because cinnamic acid (and also myrrh) has antibacterial effects. The Israelites and others used cinnamon and cassia in religious ceremonies, while in Mexico, Asiatic countries, Arabia and North Africa, it was valued in cooking. The Roman Empire imported huge amounts of cinnamon, and it may have been used mostly in perfumes and fragrances and to flavor wines, but it was not favored as a cooking spice. In the Middle Ages and subsequently, cinnamon was imported from Egypt, having been brought there by Arabian traders who obtained it in Ceylon. It became a favorite flavor in many banquet foods and was regarded as an appetite stimulator, a digestive, an aphrodisiac, and a treatment for coughs and sore throats."[10]

400 B.C.E.

Leaves of **beets** (chard) are mentioned both by Aristotle and Theophrastus. It appears that the ancients ate the leaf for food and used the root primarily as medicine, at least until the second and third centuries C.E., at which time Romans write about cooking the root of the *Beta vulgaris* (the common beet) in recipes. "The wild beet occurs widely over the Mediterranean lands, Asia Minor, the Caucasus, and the Near East. It is believed to have originated in the Mediterranean area, spreading eastward in prehistoric times, with a secondary region of development in the Near East."[11]

372 B.C.E.

The Birthday of Theophrastus. He was a significant Greek naturalist philosopher who studied with Aristotle. He wrote many treatises on plants, only two of which survive.

350 B.C.E.

Archestratus writes *Hedypatheia* (*Pleasant Living*), one of the earliest cookbooks, mentioned by Athenaeus.

Second century B.C.E.

Athenaeus, a Greek gourmet, writes *Deipnosophistai* (*The Learned Banquet*), a dialogue between two banqueters who discuss food and recipes over a period of several days.

First century C.E.

The world's oldest surviving cookbook, *De re coquinaria* (*On Cookery*), is attributed to the first century Roman, Apicius (Apicio). He documents **Pasta** using the word *lágana*, from which we get the word *lasagna*. Etruscan archaeological findings near Rome show stucco reliefs of several tools used for making these flour-based dried noodles, which predate Marco Polo's Oriental voyages.

First century C.E.

Chestnuts are eaten by the Hellenes and their descendants: "In the mountainous areas of the Mediterranean where cereals would not grow well, if at all, the chestnut (*Castanea sativa*) has been a staple food for thousands of years (Jalut 1976). Ancient Greeks and Romans, such as Dioscorides and Galen, wrote of the flatulence produced by a diet that centered too closely on chestnuts and commented on the nuts' medicinal properties, which supposedly protected against such health hazards as poisons, the bite of a mad dog, and dysentery."[12]

First century C.E.

The first mechanical dough mixer was supposedly invented by Marcus Virgilius Euryasaces, a freed slave. It "consisted of a large stone basin in which wooden paddles, powered by a horse or donkey walking in circles, kneaded the dough mixture of flour, leaven, and water." (Encyclopedia Britannica)

55 C.E.

Garlic is long considered a super food. In ancient Greece, Dioscorides (*De Materia Medica*) claimed that garlic was excellent for cleaning out arteries and opening obstructions. However, he did warn that, if used in excess, it would stir up lust and provoke lechery. This would be a concern about garlic for many centuries to come.[13]

123 C.E.

By 600 B.C. Ayurvedic physicians had identified the clinical symptoms of diabetes, blaming the condition on "dietary indiscretion." Around 400 B.C. an Indian physician named Susruta suggested that diabetes might be linked to an excess of sugar, flour, and rice in the diet.

Recommendations in the Caraka Samhita, circa 123 C.E., were for a moderate diet high in fiber and low in simple carbohydrates to counter these excesses.[14]

170 C.E.

Athenagorous, a Greek Platonist who converted to Christianity, became an important early–century Church leader and is possibly best known for his role in assuring that marine species of fish were proper dietary items for Christians. Athenagorous presented positive, counter arguments to the ideas that marine food was somehow sinful, and concluded that the Christian faithful were allowed to dine on Mediterranean fish.[15]

220 C.E.

What appears to be a recipe for **tofu** and **soymilk** is discovered on a stone slab mural during the 1980's in Henan Province, northern China. The timeline this would corroborate would be during the later Han period, 25–220 C.E. This is the oldest mention of a culinary soy preparation.

250 C.E.

Mesoamerican culture discovers the cacao bean; an early form of **chocolate** is born. The earliest records show the Mayans during the Classic Period (250–900 C.E.) using the bean (called *xoatl*), harvesting, roasting, fermenting, and grinding the seeds into paste. They did not sweeten it with cane sugar but occasionally with honey, and often took it as a bitter, medicinal drink, mixed with water and sometimes chili pepper. Later, during the time of the Aztecs, Cortez discovered the little dark beans being used as money.

Second century C.E.

The use of **Sushi** is cited in writing. "Sushi is mentioned for the first time in a dictionary compiled in China at the end of the second century A.D. It was salted fish meat in rice and was eaten after it was allowed to ferment. It is not clear whether the rice was unpolished or polished as it is now. It appears that in those days only fish meat was eaten, with the rice being discarded. So far as the history of sushi is concerned, it is certain that sushi made its debut earlier in China than in Japan. It is believed that sushi was introduced into Japan in about the seventh century A.D., though the exact date is not clear."[16]

Circa 400 C.E.

Anthimus, a fifth century Greek physician, wrote a tract entitled *The Dietetics* in which he advised Christians to be moderate in eating and drinking, and argued that foods selected should be easily and readily digestible.

He warned Christians against eating eight items: bacon rind, cheese (especially aged varieties), eggs (hard boiled), fish (old fish), mushrooms, oysters, pickled meat, and pigeon.[17]

408 C.E.

The Visigoths attack Rome and demand 3,000 pounds of pepper as part of the city's ransom.

Seventh century

Spinach predates Popeye in the Near and Far East: "Spinach is native to Iran

(Persia) and adjacent areas. It apparently was unknown outside its native land until about the beginning of the Christian era. Even then it was unknown to the Greeks and Romans. The earliest record of spinach is in Chinese, stating that it was introduced into China from Nepal 647 C.E. Old writings indicate that it reached Spain about 1100 C.E., having been brought from North Africa by the Moors. They in turn probably got it by way of ancient Syria and Arabia."[18]

Circa 800 C.E.

Legend has it that an Ethiopian goatherd discovered **coffee** beans after eating the same shrub fruit his goats were delighted by. It is the Arabs of North Africa and beyond that are credited with the discovery of roasting and brewing of the world's most popular caffeinated food. By 1000 C.E. this had become an established tradition of the Muslims, and where the Muslims went, coffee went as well. This highly prized bean did not make its way out of Africa and the Middle East until the 1600s.[19]

800 C.E.

The Chinese Cha'an (Zen) Buddhist monk Lu Yu writes the first definitive treatise on **tea**.

900 C.E.

Fish are being farm raised in China.

900 C.E.

Bananas make their way to Europe from the maritime trade routes, although they had been in long use by the people of the Indo–Malaysian region and, subsequently, the Australians.

965 C.E.

The use of **tofu** is first mentioned in writing in China in the *Chi'ng I Lu* by T'ao Ku. It was referred to as the "vice mayor's mutton," meaning the poor man's mutton, as it was likely much less expensive than meat.

1135 C.E.

King Henry I of England (1068–1135) dies, allegedly from indigestion caused by eating moray eel. Yes, he died from his eel-gotten gains.

Circa twelfth century

The notable thirteenth century medieval text, *Regimen Sanitatis Salernitanum*, a combination of Christian and Muslim dietary traditions, considers food prejudices and taboos. Included are statements on a wide range of dietary issues. Foods to be particularly avoided are those that promote the formation of black bile, while other foods are described as "enemies of the sick," and to be avoided by Christians. Examples are apple, cheese, goat, hare, meat (salted), milk, peach, pear, veal, and venison.[20]

Circa thirteenth century

The Mongolian and Turkic tribes known as the Tartars used to shred low quality Asian beef to help increase its digestibility. Steak tartar comes from this tradition—raw meat in small, thin slices. The Russian Tartars, and likely other traveling Baltic peoples, familiarize the Germans with this cuisine before the fourteenth century. Being flavored with regional spices, the Germans ate it both raw and cooked, and the poorer classes in Hamburg would make it a regular addition to the table. It became known as *Hamburg steak*, and much later in America, fried ground beef on bread would take the name **hamburger** and be a weight-inducing Big MacWhopper of a hit.

1272 C.E.

The coronation feast of King Edward I of England (1239–1307, ruled 1272–1307) included 278 bacon hogs, 450 pigs, 440 oxen, 430 sheep, and 22,600 hens and capons, although we are not sure what the guests ate.

1390

The oldest surviving cookbook in English: *The Forme of Cury.*

1411

Charles VI of France gives sole rights to the aging of Roquefort cheese to the village of Roquefort–sur–Soulzon, and all Roquefort must still be aged in these caves today.

Circa 1500

Paracelsus, the legendary Swiss physician, proposed that improper diet had a part to play in disease, challenging the Galenic notion that related it to an imbalance of the humours.[21]

1516

Duke Wilhelm IV of Bavaria decrees that

beer can only be brewed from barley malt, hops, and water. This *Rheinheitsgebot* (purity law) is the world's first consumer protection law.

1544

The existence of **tomatoes** in Italy is documented in a manuscript describing culture and herbal species of the region. "Although it is unclear where tomatoes may have been first domesticated, the two main possibilities are Peru and Mexico. The wild forms may have originated in either area, but it was the indigenous peoples of Mexico who first cultivated them. In fact, the common name *tomato* comes from *tomatl*, the word for this plant in the Nahuatl language of Mexico (Heiser 1969). Vernon Quinn proposes that the Spanish explorers brought it back to Spain from Mexico and that a Moor brought it to Tangiers, and from there, an Italian brought it to Italy where it was called Moor's apple, *pomo dei mori*, and a name with a similar sound, *poma amoris*, but a different meaning: love apple. Similarly, the French referred to it as a love apple, *pomme d'amour* (Heiser 1969)."[22]

1550

Allegedly, the first cafe in the world opens in Constantinople.

1550

Luigi Cornaro writes an autobiographical account, *Discourses on a Sober and Temperate Life*. His *Discourses* recounted a man, whose indulgencies had lead to extreme ill health by the age of forty. "Warned by physicians that he would have to trim his sails or die, Cornaro immediately converted to a programme of extreme moderation, allowing himself only twelve ounces of food and fourteen ounces of wine daily." According to Cornaro, abstinence relieved him of his ailments and renewed his vitality. He began writing *Discourses* when he was 83. They were completed when he was in his nineties.[23]

1555

Nostradamus (1503–1566) is best known for his book of prophecies *Centuries Asrtologiques,* published in 1555. However, in the same year he also published *Excellent er Moult Utile Opuscule a tous necessaire qui desirent avoir connaissance de plusieurs exquises recettes* ("An excellent and most useful little work essential to all who wish to become acquainted with some exquisite recipes").

1600

The blood orange is believed to have developed by natural mutation in Sicily.

1609

Colonial American's earliest account of the Northeast Native Tribe's use of maple syrup. The European settlers would learn how to gather this sweet sap from the American Indian's customs. Much of the early colonists' knowledge of indigenous North American medicinal plants is borrowed from the healing traditions of Native Americans.

1611	The first dairy cows are brought to Jamestown, Virginia.
1615	Venice Italy receives Europe's first shipment of green coffee beans. (The first coffee house, Caffè Florian, subsequently opens for business in 1683.)
1616	Nicholas Culpepper was born. He was an Herbalist who wrote the pseudoscientific *A Physical Directory* in 1649. It listed plants and their assumed healing properties based on the plant's resemblance to human body parts. Culpepper's influence would affect many generations of herbologists.
1670	At Cologne Cathedral, the choirmaster makes sugar sticks to give to the young singers in the choir to keep them occupied during the Living Crèche ceremony. The first **candy canes** were created. We can assume the concert was a sweet success.
1674	Jethro Tull is born: an English agriculturalist and inventor whose ideas were instrumental in the development of modern English agriculture. One of his inventions was a horse-drawn seed planting drill that sowed three even rows of seeds at once (1701). He lives an exceedingly long time and records some 36 albums, fusing madrigals with progressive English rock. He looks surprisingly well for his age.

1676	The Compagnie de Limonadiers forms in Paris. The vendors sold lemonade from tanks they carried on their backs—the first soft drinks.
1719	The first potato planted in the United States is planted in Londonderry Common Field, New Hampshire.
1734	The English author George Cheyne writes *The English Malady,* which is critical of the lifestyle of the new affluent classes that he regards as embracing excess. The expansion of trade routes also leads to the introduction of new foods and spices that he sees as being too rich for the English palate.[24]
1747	The oldest cattle ranch in the U.S. is started at Montauk on Long Island, New York.
1758	*The Compleat Housewife, or Accomplish'd Gentlewoman's Companion* by Eliza Smith is the first cookbook published in America (Williamsburg, Virginia), although written in London.[25] This is a remarkable account of the labor and knowledge required to prepare meals in an era without running water, electricity, and modern stoves.
1765	The very first pâté de foie gras (goose liver paste) is said to have been created in Strasbourg this year by a Norman chef named Jean-Joseph Close (although the technique for producing foie gras goes

back as far as the ancient Egyptians).

1773

Benjamin Delessert is born, the French industrialist who develops the first successful process for extracting sugar from sugar beets.

1789

Thomas Jefferson brings a pasta-making machine back with him when he returns to America after serving as ambassador to France.

1790

Investigation into scurvy by James Lind results in the inclusion of citrus juice in the rations of sailors in the British Navy. Although the effectiveness of citrus fruits and fresh vegetables as a cure for the disease had been reported on occasions throughout the seventeenth century, it was not until the 1790s that this became British Navy policy.[26]

1820

The first compendium of standard drugs in the U.S. is established with the U.S. Pharmacopeia when 11 physicians meet in Washington, D.C.

1823

A Frenchman, Count Odette Phillipe, plants the first grapefruit trees in Florida around Tampa Bay. Today, Florida produces more grapefruit than the rest of the world combined.

1824

John Simpson Chisum is born, American frontiersman and cattle rancher. In 1867 he blazed the Chisum Trail from Paris, Texas, to Fort Sumner, New Mexico. Between 1870 and 1881 he had the largest cattle herd in the U.S. near Roswell, New Mexico. Perhaps this is why aliens were alleged to have visited there—the odds were in their favor for locating a choice patty melt.

1824

Ferdinand Carre is born, a French engineer and pioneer in refrigeration methods. In 1859 he invents the ammonia vapor–compression system that becomes the most widely used at the time. Vapor compression is still the system most in use today.

1828

The word *cupcake* is first found in *Receipts* by E. Leslie.

1828

C.J. Van Houten of the Netherlands develops Dutch–process cocoa (**cocoa powder**). Cold winter days will be just a little more bearable.

1829

Sylvester Graham invents the **Graham cracker**.

1834

The first U.S. patent for a refrigerating machine is issued. Jacob Perkins patents a refrigerating machine that uses sulphuric ether compression.

1845

Peter Cooper, inventor and founder of the Cooper Union for the Advancement of

Science and Art, obtains the first American patent for the manufacture of gelatin. In 1895, cough syrup manufacturer Pearl B. Wait purchases the patent and develops a packaged gelatin dessert. Wait's wife, May David Wait, names it **Jell-O**.

1846 Nancy Johnson invents the hand-cranked ice cream freezer. Nothing more is known about her. In 1848, William G. Young patents her design.

1847 Purportedly, Captain Hanson Gregory originates the hole in the center of the doughnut. He uses the top of a round tin pepper container to punch the holes, so the dough would cook evenly.

1848 Pasta is produced commercially in the U.S. for the first time.

1848 Throughout the eighteenth and nineteenth centuries, people believed that eating fresh fruit caused serious illness, even death. During the cholera epidemic of 1848, the *Chicago Daily Journal* spread a fear of orchard-grown produce. Still another report claimed that a man who simply passed a fruit stand filled with spoiled peaches suffered a severe attack of the "gripes." Panic ensued, and people refused to eat fruit even after it was proven that the link between peaches and cholera was not the fruit itself but the fruit-sellers' habit of washing their produce in polluted streams. This fear of fruit continued for many years.[27]

1849

Self-service restaurants first appear in San Francisco during the California gold rush of 1849. At first a selection of free food was placed along the bar in saloons. There were so many people that other businesses soon opened and charged for self-serving. You went down the line with a tray, picked what you wanted, and paid at the end of the line. Regrettably, anti-bacterial soap and sneeze guards would not be invented for 125 years.

1850

The American Vegetarian Society is founded.

Mid 1800s

Devotees of the poet Byron (George Gordon, 1788–1824) adopt his horror of fat as symbolizing dullness and lethargy. According to the American writer George Beard, "Our young ladies live all their growing girlhood in semi-starvation" because of a fear of "incurring the horror of the disciples of Lord Byron."[28]

1851

Dr. John Gorrie of Apalachicola, Florida, is granted the first U.S. patent for mechanical refrigeration in 1851.

1851

In Baltimore, Jacob Fussell establishes the first **commercial ice cream** plant.

1862

President Lincoln appoints a chemist,

Charles M. Wetherill, to serve in the new Department of Agriculture. This is the beginning of the Bureau of Chemistry, the predecessor of the Food and Drug Administration[29].

1863

Granula, probably the **first breakfast cereal**, is introduced. Dr. James C. Jackson of Dansville, N.Y., created it.

1869

Joseph Campbell, a fruit merchant, and Abram Anderson, an icebox maker, get together to can tomatoes, vegetables, fruit preserves, etc. This is the beginning of the Campbell Soup Company.

1870

Ellen White and husband set up Battle Creek Sanatorium. In 1876, John Harvey Kellogg (who later invents Corn Flakes) takes up the position of medical director. Under Kellogg's direction, the clients, in addition to being offered diet–based health regimes, are subjected to enemas, bed rest, hydrotherapy, and exercise.

1871

Luther Burbank develops the Russet Burbank potato, near Santa Rosa, California. He becomes celebrated for his ingenuity in hybrids and plant modifications.

1871

Charles Feltman, a German butcher, opens up the first Coney Island hot dog stand, selling 3,684 dachshund sausages (now called **hot dogs**) in a milk roll during his first year in business.

1871

Thomas Adams patents a chewing–gum–producing machine. He manufactures the first commercially successful chewing gum, Black Jack.

1872

Walter Scott of Providence, Rhode Island, invents the horse drawn lunch wagon. The prototypical meals–on–wheels truck is born.

1872

Henry Tate, an English sugar merchant, patents a method of cutting sugar into small cubes in 1872. He makes a fortune and so will the healthcare industry.

1873

Mr. Adolphus Busch develops a method of pasteurizing beer so it can withstand temperature fluctuations, which enables national distribution.

1880

The wholesale price of lobster is 10 cents per pound, close to $2.00 a pound in today's money, revealing that it has always been pricey.

1881

Dr. Satori Kato of Japan introduces the first instant coffee at the Pan American World Fair. The American coffee giant Starbucks would reciprocate the favor in August of 1996 by opening its first of 500 Japanese outlets in Tokyo's Ginza district.

1882

Swiss flour manufacturer Julius Maggi begins commercial production of the first bouillon cubes. He develops them so the poor have a cheap method for making nutritious soup.

1884 Dr. Hervey D. Thatcher, of Potsdam, New York, invents the milk bottle.

1885 Philadelphia brand cream cheese goes on sale; cheesecake and at-home weighing devices follow.

1885 Dr Pepper is invented in Waco, Texas. There is no period after the "Dr" in Dr Pepper; there is no pepper, either.

1885 Some historians describe the decades surrounding the turn of the century as the golden age of food faddism. Vociferous vegetarians did battle with ardent meat eaters in an attempt to gain the moral and scientific high ground on all things relating to diet. Also competing were the no-breakfast faddists, the raw-food faddists, and those who refused to contemplate any food that was fermented. Often their strict regimes were supported by their own personal struggles with poor health. Yes, some things never change.[30]

1887 Asa Candler (1851–1929), a wholesale druggist, purchases the formula for Coca-Cola from John S. Pemberton, an Atlanta pharmacist, for $2,300. He sold the company in 1919 for $25 million.

1889 Aunt Jemima Pancake mix is introduced.

It is the first ready-mix food to be sold commercially; more at-home weighing devices will be sold.

1891

Fig Newtons are created by Kennedy Biscuit Works in Cambridgeport, Massachusetts.

1893

Dachshund Sausages become the standard fare at baseball parks (later, **hot dogs**). This tradition was probably started by a St. Louis bar owner, Chris Von de Ahe, a German immigrant who also owned the St. Louis Browns major league baseball team.

1895

Postum cereal beverage introduced by Postum Cereal Co.

1895

Rudolph Boysen is born. He developed the boysenberry, a raspberry-blackberry hybrid in 1923.

1895

Gennaro Lombardi opens the first pizzeria in the U.S. in New York City. (Some other sources say it was 1905.)

1896

Leo Hirshfield of New York introduces Tootsie Rolls, named after his daughter's nickname, Tootsie.

1898

Caleb D. Bradham, a New Bern, North Carolina pharmacist, creates Pepsi-Cola, in imitation of Coca-Cola. (He originally called it Brad's Drink.) Let the wars for profit begin.

1900   Hershey's Milk Chocolate Bar is created.

1902   In the early years of the twentieth cen-
                            tury, William Hay introduced the notion
                            of food combining. Hay believed that
                            toxins and accumulated waste in the
                            body caused disease. The Hay diet advo-
                            cated the avoidance of "foods that fight."
                            For example, carbohydrates should not
                            be combined with proteins in the same
                            meal, and foods should be consumed that
                            restore the natural acid–alkaline balance
                            in our bodies. The Hay Diet will experi-
                            ence a particularly high profile resur-
                            gence in 1991, when it will be widely
                            reported that the Duchess of Kent is ad-
                            hering to it.[31]

1902   The National Biscuit Company changes
                            the name of their Animal Biscuits to
                            Barnum's Animals and redesigns the
                            package as a circus wagon with a string
                            attached so it can be hung on Christmas
                            trees. They sell for 5 cents a box.

1902   The pastel–colored candy disks called
                            NECCO wafers first appear, named for the
                            New **E**ngland **C**onfectionery **Co**mpany.

1903   First U.S. patent for instant coffee.

1904   George J. French introduces **French's
                            mustard** the same year the hot dog is
                            introduced to America at the St. Louis
                            World's Fair. Baseball parks would soon

bring the two products together in an inseparable wedding of American culinary matrimony.

1904   Thomas Sullivan of New York City invents the **tea bag**. He first uses them to send tea samples to his customers, instead of sending them in more expensive tins.

1904   **Puffed Rice** is introduced at the St. Louis World's Fair. It was developed by Dr. Alexander P. Anderson of New York City, and first manufactured by American Cereal Co. (which later becomes the Quaker Oats Co).

1904   **Post Toasties** are introduced by General Foods (originally called Elijah's Manna.)

1904   R. Blechyden serves tea with ice at the St. Louis World's Fair and invents **iced tea**.

1904   The **ice cream cone** is invented at the St. Louis World's Fair. An ice cream vendor ran out of paper cups and asked a nearby waffle booth to make some thin waffles he could roll up to hold the ice cream.

1904   John D. Rockefeller, eminent industrialist and entrepreneur, declares that he has conquered a serious illness by reducing the amount of food that he eats.

1905   Frank Epperson invents **popsicles** in 1905; they were originally called *Epsicles*.

1905

Upton Sinclair writes *The Jungle*, a grim indictment of the meat–packing industry, which leads to national outrage and government reforms of the food industry.

1906

The Food and Drug Act of 1906 is signed by Theodore Roosevelt, paving the way for the first full reforms of dangers in the commercial food supply.

1907

One of the ad campaigns for Kellogg's Corn Flakes (then the Battle Creek Toasted Corn Flake Company) offers a free box of cereal to every woman who will wink at her grocer. The grocers are happy.

1911

Hereward Carrington's 1908 book *Vitality, Fasting and Nutrition* recommends regular fasting for good health. Upton Sinclair (1878–1968) follows up on Carrington's theory in 1911 with his own book, *The Fasting Cure*, which recommends long periods of starvation as a means of combating tuberculosis, syphilis, asthma, liver trouble, and cancer.[32]

1912

Richard Hellmann, a New York deli owner, created his recipe for bottled **mayonnaise** in 1903. He begins to market it this year.

1914

In U.S. v. Lexington Mill and Elevator Company, the Supreme Court issues its first ruling on food additives. It is ruled that in order for bleached flour with nitrate residues to be banned from foods, the government must show a relationship between the chemical additive and the harm it is to allegedly cause in humans. The court also noted that the mere presence of such an ingredient was not sufficient to render the food illegal.

1914

James L. Kraft founds the J. L. Kraft Bros. cheese factory in Stockton, Illinois.

1916

Electric refrigerators are first offered for sale at $900. Just as a comparison, a Model-T Ford in 1927 sells for $650. With adjustments for inflation, a standard refrigerator would be approximately $23,000 today.

1921

Advertising manager Sam Gale of General Mills invents Betty Crocker.

1927

Edwin E. Perkins of Hastings, Nebraska, invents the powdered soft drink Kool-Aid.

1929

7-Up is invented and originally called Bib-Label Lithiated Lemon-Lime Soda, something you cannot order in a hurry.

1936

Robert Cobb invents the Cobb salad at his Brown Derby Restaurant in Hollywood, California.

1937

Spam is developed by George A. Hormel & Co. and first marketed in 1937. Monty Python fans rejoice in retrospect.

1937	Kraft Macaroni & Cheese is introduced: "Make a meal in 9 minutes or less for 19 cents or less."
1937	107 people are killed, mostly children, by elixir of sulfanilamide, which contains the poisonous solvent diethylene glycol. This magnifies the need to establish food additive safety before marketing and persuades Congress to pass the pending revision of the 1906 Food and Drugs Act, the revised rendition of which was introduced in 1933.
1938	The Federal Food, Drug, and Cosmetic (FDC) Act is passed by Congress with new legal provisions, including "safe tolerance levels for unavoidable poisonous substances," and requirement for new drugs to be proven safe before marketing the chemical.
1939	The seedless watermelon is developed.
1940	The first Dairy Queen opens in Joliet, Illinois. They will grow to 5,900 facilities in the U.S. and Canada, with 20 overseas outlets.
1943	The USDA releases its "Seven Basic Food Groups" in the National Wartime Nutrition Guide. This will later be trimmed to four.
1946	Tupperware is launched.

1948	Ultra–high temperature pasteurization is introduced for commercial milk.
1950	Frank McNamara creates the first credit card, the Diners Club, as a result of forgetting his wallet after dining at a restaurant.
1950	Pillsbury launches its annual bake–off to promote its flour.
1950	The Open Kettle, a coffee and donut shop in Quincy, Massachusetts, is renamed Dunkin' Donuts. The first franchise is sold in 1955.
1950	Minute Rice is introduced.
1950	During this year, an American doctor, John Gofman, puts forward a hypothesis that blood cholesterol is to blame for the rise in coronary heart disease. This is supported in 1951 when pathologists are sent to Korea to learn about war wounds by dissecting the bodies of dead soldiers. To their surprise, they discover unexpected evidence of coronary heart disease—unexpected because they knew that death from heart disease was extremely rare under middle age, and these men averaged only twenty–two years of age. So the pathologists performed detailed dissections on the hearts of the next 300 corpses. In 35% they found deposits of fibrous, fatty material sticking to the artery

walls. A further 41% had fully formed lesions, and in 3% of the soldiers these lesions were sufficiently large that they blocked at least one coronary artery. Thus, over three-quarters of all the men examined showed evidence of serious coronary heart disease—and they were barely out of their teens."[33]

1951

Gerber Products starts using MSG (monosodium glutamate) in its baby foods to make them taste better.

1952

Kellogg's Cereal introduces Sugar Frosted Flakes, 29% sugar.

1952

Howard Johnson's becomes the world's largest food chain when it opens its 351st restaurant. The growing fast-food movement would displace HoJo's restaurant glory 27 years later when the British company Imperial Group PLC would purchase them in September of 1979.

1953

Dow Chemical creates Saran Wrap

1953

Sugar Smacks are introduced, containing 56% sugar.

1954

M&M's Peanut Chocolate Candies are introduced. Also, the famous slogan "The milk chocolate melts in your mouth, not in your hand" is started.

1954

Let's Eat Right to Keep Fit by Adele Davis is

published, one of the earlier health food books.

1954

Trix cereal is introduced by General Mills. It is more than 46% sugar.

1956

80% of U.S. households have a refrigerator, compared to only 8% of British households.

1957

Margarine sales exceed butter for the first time.

1958

The Food Additives Amendment is initiated, requiring manufacturers of new food additives to establish safety prior to marketing. The Delaney proviso prohibits the approval of any food additive shown to promote cancer in humans or animals. This same year, the FDA publishes in the Federal Register the first list of substances Generally Recognized as Safe (GRAS), which contains nearly 200 substances.[34]

1958

Cocoa Puffs is created by General Mills; it contains 43% sugar.

1958

Cocoa Krispies is created by Kellogg's, with 45.9% sugar.

1958

There are 4,063 drive-in movie screens nationwide. A fourth of the automobiles will drive away with the speaker still attached to the window.

1958	Jolly Green Giant is born. He appears on TV but looks like a monster and scares children. In response, the Green Giant Company lightens him up a bit, adds "Ho, ho, ho" and a catchy jingle. We should have listened to the children.
1959	There are 32,000 supermarkets in the U.S., which account for 69% of all food store sales.
1960	"The term *lifestyle* emerged during the 1960s to describe the way an individual chose certain behaviors that predisposed them to illness. *Lifestyle* also implies that personal habits are discrete and in-dependently modifiable, that individuals could voluntarily choose to alter certain behaviors, and that each person has a re-sponsibility for living well through self-discipline and behavior modification."[35]
1961	A technique for tenderizing beef is pat-ented. It involves injecting papain, an enzyme made from papaya, directly into the bloodstream of living animals. PETA would not be created for another 29 years.
1962	President John F. Kennedy proclaims the **Consumer Bill of Rights** to Congress. Included are the right to safety, the right to be informed, the right to choose, and the right to be heard.
1963	Irradiation is applied for the first time to

sterilize dried fruits and vegetables.

1964   The first 12-ounce aluminum can is introduced by Royal Crown Cola. It is not until 3 years later that Coke starts using the aluminum can.

1965   Cool Whip, a whipped cream substitute, is introduced by General Foods.

1967   Gatorade, the original sports drink, is developed by the University of Florida for their football team.

1967   Wisconsin is the last state to allow coloring to be added to margarine.

1970   In *Upjohn v. Finch*, the Court of Appeals upholds enforcement of the 1962 drug effectiveness amendments by ruling that commercial success alone does not constitute substantial evidence of drug safety and efficacy.

1973   Nathaniel Weyth receives a patent for PET (polyethylene terephthalate) beverage bottles. This is the first safe plastic strong enough to hold carbonated beverages without bursting. Soda in plastic bottles would soon fill supermarket shelves.

1974   Pop Rocks are revealed by General Foods. Ever since 1956, when company research chemist William Mitchell found a way to put carbon dioxide into a solid, General

Foods searched for a way to market the invention. The popping, crackling candy turns out to be worth the wait; in only five years the company will have sold 500 million packets of Pop Rocks.

1978

Ben & Jerry's Homemade Ice Cream and Crepes opens in Burlington, Vermont, at a gas station on the corners of St. Paul and College streets with a $12,000 investment. They post a net sales earning of over $237 million dollars for 1999, with a Unilever Corporate buy-out of $326 million dollars in 2000.

1981

The FDA approves the artificial sweetener aspartame. There has been a litany of controversy over the safety of this product ever since[36].

1982

Newman's Own Food is founded by Paul Newman, a company that devotes all profits to charity—over $100 million to over 1,000 charities. Humanists worldwide thank Mr. Newman.

1985

"Although hunger in a world of plenty is a tale as old as time, the contrast has seldom been demonstrated more graphically than it was in 1985. While the American administration sent $500 million to help save the lives of the wasted skeletons of Ethiopia, Americans themselves spent $5,000 million on trying to lose weight."[37]

1994	rBST, or recombinant Bovine Somatotropin (also marketed as Posilac or bST) is approved for commercial use in the United States as a safe and effective means to increase milk production in cows.[38] Monsanto Corporation creates it.
1995	The FDA declares cigarettes to be "drug delivery devices." Restrictions are recommended on marketing and sales to reduce smoking by young people.
1996	Olestra fat substitute is approved. Proctor and Gamble manufactures it.
1997	Congress passes The Food and Drug Modernization Act (FDAMA). This legislation provides fast-track approval of certain new drugs and accelerated approval for certain medical devices by exempting them from pre-market notification requirements.
1998	In West Virginia if you run over an animal, you can legally take it home and cook it for dinner. A law passed in 1998 lets drivers keep their road kill, as long as they report it within 12 hours. According to supporters of the new law, the state will save money that had been used to have Highway Division employees remove dead animals from the road.
2003	March: "Food combining 'fights cancer.'" Eating certain foods together, such as

chicken and broccoli or salmon and watercress could help to fight cancer, say researchers. Combining two food components called sulforaphane and selenium make them up to 13 times more powerful in attacking cancer together than they are alone, they suggested. The discovery could mean it could be possible to design special cancer–fighting foods or diets. This was originally published in the journal *Carcinogenesis*.[39]

13

Our Fast-Food Fasci-Nation

IN THE DOCUMENTARY, "SUPERSIZE ME," A HEALTHY MAN, MORGAN Spurlock, takes on an interesting experiment to make a point: eating nothing but McDonald's for one month while being monitored by three health professionals to determine if there are any physical detriments as a result of this fast–food diet. The outcome of this experiment was quite startling.

Morgan's idea was inspired by a popular news story of a reported lawsuit claiming that eating McDonald's food was detrimental to the health of the lawsuit plaintiffs. The judge in the case stated that the lawsuit would be valid only if the plaintiffs could prove an inherent danger in consuming McDonald's food. Mr. Spurlock's attitude was "Let's see," and so a documentary was born.

The movie's brave volunteer, a six–foot–two–inch, one–hundred–eighty–five–and–a–half–pound non–smoking male with 11% body fat, increases to two hundred ten pounds and 18% body fat at the end of his experiment. His caloric intake escalates from an estimated 2,500 to 5,000. His cholesterol rises from 168 to 230, and he starts exhibiting many symptoms of disease: shortness of breath, chest tightness, depression, sexual dysfunction, and lethargy, to name but a few. In the film, the cardiologist and the general practitioner both implore him to cease the experiment out of concern for the damage he seems to be doing to his heart and liver.

This is an extreme case but not one completely extraordinary in our culture. The film mentions the statistics about regular and very regular patrons of McDonald's. You may be surprised to discover how many people eat fast food three to five times a week—every week!

The amount of fast food he consumes in a month is reported to be equal to what the average person would consume in eight years. The difficult term to establish here is *average.*

This is not the only basis for our country's present obesity epidemic, but coupled with a sedentary lifestyle, it could be a significant factor.

Some other interesting information that comes from this compelling documentary:

- Fast-food portions have increased three times from the inception of the fast-food phenomenon in the late 1950s. We used to be satisfied with one-third of today's restaurant portion. Our waistlines are revealing our gluttony.
- Some 60% of Americans are either overweight or obese.
- Approximately 17 million Americans (about 1 in 20) have Type II adult-onset diabetes, which has a very strong dietary connection.
    - If a young person is diagnosed with Type II diabetes, and there is not sufficient intervention, it can take between 17 to 27 years off his or her lifespan.
    - Direct medical costs have more than doubled for Type II diabetes—$44 billion in 1997 to $92 billion in 2002.
- The average American child sees 10,000 food advertisements per year on television; 90% of these are for sugary snacks or fast food.

This is not an indictment of McDonald's; of course, the same could be said of any fast-food corporation. McD's is just the biggest and the one that the others usually try to emulate in one way or another. The arguments that could be made on behalf of the fast-food companies are these: (1) They don't expect a person to eat three meals a day at their establishments and (2) Their food is not designed to be a successful substitute for a homemade well-balanced meal.

Commonsense prevents one from suing any food establishment, fast-food or otherwise, because a person gets fat eating its food. Quite frankly, that is not the restaurant's problem. Everyone knows that most all restaurants serve food high in salt and fat—that is what appeals to our palate. We know that alcohol intoxicates us, hot coffee is hot to drink, and fast food will make us gain weight if overindulged in.

If your health is good overall, you can indulge occasionally without it being notable to any significant degree. The problem always arises when we get out of balance—when we allow extremes to continue without nipping them in the McBud.

Perhaps the most worrisome aspect of the "Supersize Me" documentary is its revelation of the eating habits of our children in school. We see how children get inculcated with messages from convenience food corporations, even at school, where there are numerous soda machines and, in some school districts, fast-food establishments on the school premises.

The film cites an example of modifying behavior through changes in diet at a school in Appleton, Wisconsin. This school for troubled teens abolished all fried foods, sodas, candy, and pre-packaged foods and instead chose a natural food company to come in to prepare the students' meals. The change in behavior was dramatic according to the school's principle.

Behavior and nutrition have been the objects of study for many years, and the data is overwhelmingly in support of real foods in place of convenience foods for developing bodies and minds. The orthomolecular nutrition pioneer, Dr. Abram Hoffer, has written extensively about his experiences in changing behavioral problems in adolescents with nutritional therapy. He advocates using vitamins and foods first for remedying ADHD, instead of dispensing Riddlin as an initial intervention. If we do not address the underlying nutritional causes of the dysfunction but instead add powerful chemicals into a young person's already chemically imbalanced system, we create a recipe for tragic consequences. This same concept applies to adults.

What we eat affects us physically and emotionally. Watching Morgan Spurlock go through his transformations from health to disease is a revealing glimpse into how excess exerts a high toll upon both body and mind. Keeping indulgences in fast food and sweets to a minimum may be one of the wisest restrictions of all. You cannot talk people out of their bad eating habits, but let them suffer long enough and perhaps through their own disease they will be motivated enough to change. When the diner is ready, the veggies will appear.

14

Food Additives

"Nearly 15,000 substances are added to the foods we eat during their growth, processing, and packaging. These additives are subjected to extremely careful laboratory screening before they are used, and scientists believe it is unlikely that they contribute significantly to the overall cancer risk in humans."[1]

THE BUSINESS OF FOOD IS A BIG BUSINESS—ONE OF THE MOST POWerful lobbyist organizations in the country. The big money that the food giants spend to influence legislation in their favor affects the average consumer in numerous ways, some positive, and some not-so positive.

Let's face it; it is a difficult endeavor to feed 295,166,191[2] people, not counting our food industry exports. Mass-marketing food products that used to be available in our own backyards or just down the road at the local farm comes with numerous difficulties.

The food companies have to make the food product look appealing in a static and packaged state; they need to make sure the product lasts long enough to get to the grocery distributor and remain on the shelf without expiring; they need to ensure that the texture and consistency is reminiscent of something cooked in a home or professional kitchen; they need to compensate for the lack of natural flavors and aromas in stored, synthetic, and processed food products. In short, the business of food is the business of sales—they need to create a convincing illusion for you to buy.

We could think of the food industry as a hybrid of the fashion and cosmetics industries with a smooth creamy filling of the pharmaceutical industry added for extra enjoyment. This business is edible fashion, ingestible make–up, and "safe" chemical enhancement. For the status quo, whatever doesn't kill you (at least not provable in a court of law) makes the food giants more affluent.

No one is calling the food business the "health business." If our present health system were based on the ethics of the Chinese of antiquity, wherein the physician was paid only if his patient got better or remained disease free, we might be able to call the medical profession the health profession. We seem to have developed a preoccupation with disease, with hundreds of ways to inform the consumer about being ill and very few ways to define health and wellness; just how do you know you are healthy?

There seems to be a schism between people who are health oriented and people who take a live–and–let–live, devil-may–care attitude about health. After all, we have these lunatic fringe storehouses with the puzzling name of "health food stores" that "health nuts" patronize if they want something that is good for them. This is not what mainstream America desires, is it? We don't really want to eat for health, do we? We would prefer something that tastes good, real good, and forces us to get on the stationary bike as a penance. Oh, forget about that; we have technology to save us: "Ten pounds of liposuction please, and make that to go." What the fried pork and mud pie giveth, the surgeon taketh away.

Food manufacturers are just filling a niche; they see a commercial need, and the free–market ships sail victoriously into the ports with the blessings of the governmental regulators. When it comes to what is in the food you eat, you must put your trust in the efficacy of reams of bureaucratic red tape and the status quo of a scientific model that too often assumes nature to be second–rate to technological prowess.

This prowess is widely exercised in the chemicalization of the food supply. The largest categories for food additives contain chemicals that achieve the objective of creating the illusion of palatability. Stabilizers keep food ingredients bound together, emulsifiers help oils and water mix together, anti-caking agents keep granulated products from clumping, and flavor enhancers render the organically pallid into the chemically fantastic. This chemical alteration of food has advanced to a stage where many young people are unfamiliar with the actual taste of a food, often a fruit, and prefer the synthesized, counterfeit version; strawberry- and grape-flavored are preferred to the actual fruit.

According to the *Canadian Journal of Orthomolecular Medicine*, "Food additives in use today can be divided roughly into three main types: cosmetics, preservatives, and processing aids, totaling presently about 3,794 different additives, of which over 3,640 are used purely as cosmetics, 63 as preservatives, and 91 as processing aids."[3] This paper states that the "Western diet . . . is made up of various processed foods" estimated to be about 75% of the average consumer's diet or about "8–10 lbs of food additives [per person] per year." The study continues with its central idea that the increase of additives in food has a significant influence on child behavior, especially childhood hyperactivity, aka Attention Deficit Hyperactivity Disorder (ADHD), Cerebral Brain Dysfunction Disorder, et al.

A rather famous report on the dangers of food additives was initiated by Dr. Benjamin F. Feingold, M.D., Chief Emeritus, Allergy Department, Kaiser Permanente Hospital, San Francisco, California, in 1964. In studying over 1,200 cases, his team found that "hyperactivity . . . [and] other neurophysiological disturbances" could be induced when some children consumed certain food additives, especially ones that contain salicylates, like those in aspirin. What is remarkable is that Dr. Feingold removed all foods with synthetic food additives, and the children's behavioral abnormalities regulated. Subsequent to this controversial study, a few researchers have refuted Dr. Feingold's findings, but their refutations have since come under scrutiny.

One of the significant food additives studied was tartrazine, which is used as a food coloring most frequently by the soft drink industry. For people who have aspirin sensitivities, "10–40% of the aspirin-sensitive patients are usually also affected by tartrazine." Besides hyperactivity, asthma was also mentioned as being a reaction to this additive. If this same reaction is present in adults, it would have substantial implications. This inflammatory reaction that causes asthmatic symptoms could be eliminated simply by removing soft drink and processed foods from the table. Who knew?

Most parents would likely take the child to a physician who would prescribe medication for the symptoms, which could never be fully effective because the child (or adult) keeps ingesting the compounds that instigate the problem. This is one way to get aboard the medication merry–go round; there are many others.

Now you may be thinking, "Just how many soft drinks would one have to consume for that reaction to occur?" Before you think of some astronomical number, the report cited " . . . an oral administration of 50 mg tartrazine to 122 patients suffering from allergy–related disorders evoked . . . the feeling of suffocation, weakness, heat sensation, palpitations, and blurred vision, to name most on the list. A few servings a day of soft drinks are all that is needed to replicate this dosage.

There have been other studies since these that corroborate the connection between tartrazine consumption and abnormal behavioral patterns. One study in 1995 found 79% corroboration in 76 children diagnosed as hyperactive.[4]

In keeping with the virtues of soft drinks, the additive usually labeled as *caramels* or *caramel coloring* is another cosmetic agent (of which over 100 caramel varieties are in use) that has been linked to "convulsions when fed to rats, mice and chicks." It also has proven adverse to the production of white blood cells and lymphocytes, both crucial components of the immune system.[5]

The two most prolific food additives in the processed American food supply are sugar and salt. If we take a brief look at refined sugar consumption, it clearly emerges as the most destructive of all food additives. Some estimates are that Americans consume 20% of the world's sugar and have every year since the Civil War. Americans diets are estimated by some sources to contain 20–35% refined sugar per meal.

You may be surprised to see how easy it is to ingest large amounts of sugar without even trying. The following accounts for a typical American day:

Food	Amount of sugar
Breakfast:	
1 piece of toasted white bread	3 teaspoons
1 bowl of presweetened breakfast cereal	3–4 teaspoons
1 6-ounce glass of orange juice	3 teaspoons
1 glazed donut	6 teaspoons
Lunch:	
1 12-ounce serving of a popular soft drink	9 teaspoons
hamburger bun	3 teaspoons
convenience-style apple pie	12 teaspoons
standard chocolate bar	7–10 teaspoons
Dinner:	
1 soda	9–14 teaspoons
TV Dinner	3–5 teaspoons
1 slice pie	10–12 teaspoons
2 slices white bread	6 teaspoons
Daily total	up to 87 teaspoons !!

Dr. John Yudkin in *Pure White and Deadly: the problem of sugar*. Davis-Poynter, London. 1972—"If only a small fraction of what is already known about the effects of sugar were to be revealed in relation to any other material used as a food additive, that material would be promptly banned."

Dr. Linus Pauling Ph.D., "The Pauling Institute Letter," Fall 1986: "Each molecule of sucrose is converted to one molecule of glucose and one of fructose. Glucose is metabolized as a source of energy, but the metabolism of fructose produces acetate, which is involved in the formation of cholesterol."

There are many reasons to read the ingredients in your favorite foods. The following three additives are among the most problematic with numerous reported sensitivities:

1. *Refined Cane Sugar*

There is no doubt here. This is clearly one of the most hazardous chemicals in the commercial food system. What makes it most insidious is its wide acceptance as a harmless inert product. If you would ingest it in small doses on a very irregular basis, and your health were good, you would likely have no worse effects from refined sugar than from breathing in carbon monoxide in fifteen minutes of rush hour traffic. This would not be a nontoxic effect but a relatively negligible one. The problem is that sugar is in virtually everything, and it is consumed in excessive amounts at every occasion, in every restaurant, and at every event across the country; akin to spending eight hours a day breathing in the traffic's exhaust.

Two intriguing studies in the late 1980s link refined sugar consumption to significant incidences of criminal and antisocial behavior.[6] One study tested 276 incarcerated juvenile offenders by substituting sugary drinks and foods and junk food snacks with more healthful choices such as fruit juices, nuts, and fresh fruits. As a result, assault and battery dropped by 82%, theft by 77%, and refusal–to–obey–orders by 55%. Parents today think they need Dr. Phil for their disciplinary challenges when it may be as simple as cleaning out the junk foods and introducing real foods. Another study of 1,382 juveniles showed a drop in rule violations by 25% in just 3 months by eliminating refined sugar products. Another study, including 2,005 offenders, showed a 21% decrease in rule violations, 25% decrease in assaults and fights, and a 42% diminishment in general disruptions. Every correctional facility and high school in the country would pine for those numbers.

These studies and at least 25 years of research on the negative health effects of refined sugar win it the #1 position for most problematic food additive.

2. *Artificial Sweeteners*

Aspartame is a prime offender and is found in many artificially sweetened products. The key ingredient is phenylalanine, an amino acid that is commonly used by soft drink and convenience food purveyors. At least in rat experiments, "aspartame was found to double the level of phenylalaline in their brains, which redoubled when other carbohydrates were consumed at the same time." The "other carbohydrates" applicable to human's food consumption could be potato chips, pretzels, cheese puffs, and popcorn, many of the snack foods that commonly accompany soda consumption.

Eventually a neurochemical chain reaction occurs in this experiment, depleting serotonin levels in the rats. Serotonin is a powerful neurochemical associated with moods, emotions, appetite, and sleep. Serotonin retention is a key clinical focus to counteracting diagnosed clinical depression. A reduction or imbalance of serotonin in the brain has many implications: aggression, depression, and manic behavior are just a few.

Aspartame has had a litany of complaints filed against it to the FDA. There appear to be an above-average number of side-effect complaints associated with Aspartame consumption. Perhaps you are among the percentage of consumers who have no measurable side-effects. If not, you are well-advised to change your product consumption.

3. *High-Fructose Corn Syrup*

Have you tried lately to buy sweetened food products that are not made with high-fructose corn syrup? Have you noticed how many pre-packaged foods contain HFCS? It is very difficult to locate HFCS-free products in most national chain supermarkets. Why are products sweetened with HFCS problematic? Here are a few items to consider:

1. According to Linda Joyce Forristal, writing for the Weston A. Price Foundation, "Today Americans consume more HFCS than sugar."[7] The regular consumption of refined sugar has its own detriments to the body, but HFCS appears to have even more. HFCS is essentially a chemical transformation of cornstarch into a clear white

sweetener that is one-and-a-half times as sweet as standard sucrose (table sugar). According to Ms. Forristal, HFCS, compared to table sugar "is obviously much more complicated to make, involving vats of murky fermenting liquid, fungus, and chemical tweaking, all of which take place in one of 16 chemical plants located in the Corn Belt. Yet in spite of all the special enzymes required, HFCS is actually cheaper than sugar. It is also very easy to transport—it's just piped into tanker trucks. This translates into lower costs and higher profits for food producers."

She also asserts that most, if not all, HFCS is produced through genetic modification technology. In the process of creating a syrup from cornstarch "two of the enzymes used, alpha-amylase and glucose-isomerase, are genetically modified to make them more stable [for higher processing temperatures]." Since the four major corporations that manufacture HFCS (Archer Daniels Midland, Cargill, Staley Manufacturing Co., and CPC International) employ the same basic chemical processes, it is likely that all HFCS is the end result of genetic modification.

2. The North Carolina supermarket chain Earth Fare banned the use of HFCS according to an August 1, 2004 press release.[8] Company representatives claimed that HFCS products are "too processed and refined for their food product philosophy and given current research, does not match their 'healthy' mission." According to the press release, "High fructose corn syrup has been implicated in studies as a possible contributor to America's twin epidemics of obesity and Type II diabetes. First introduced into the American diet in mass quantities in the 1970s, its introduction was followed by the rapid rise in Type II diabetes and obesity amongst Americans in the eighties and nineties. These health

crises continue to this day."

3. Meira Fields, Ph.D., a research chemist at the USDA in Beltsville, Maryland, has conducted numerous studies correlating disease and nutrition. One in particular that relates to excess fructose consumption, as in HFCS, was implemented on two groups of rats. One group was fed a low-copper, high-fructose diet and the other a low-copper, high complex-carbohydrate diet. According to Ms. Fields, "Rats normally live for a good two years, but the rats in my study fed high-fructose, low-copper diets are dying after 5 weeks." As indicated by her abstract in the *Journal of the American College of Nutrition*,[9] "For the majority of people, particularly if they do not smoke, the food they eat is the largest controllable factor determining their long-term health." She concludes her assessment of high fructose consumption with "Diets consumed in industrialized societies including the US are relatively high in simple sugars, total fat, and saturated fat. These dietary components have been known to affect the glucose/insulin system."

Although the manufacturers of HFCS insist on its safety, you may try eliminating it from your diet to see if you feel better as a result. Our food supply is inundated with this chemically mutated sweetener, one that most people's systems could do well to eliminate.

15

Phytomedicine–The Healing Power of Plants

MEDICINE, AS WE KNOW IT TODAY, HAS EVOLVED OVER HUNDREDS of years from the traditional and folk medicine usage of plants and fungi to heal ailments and strengthen the body.

> "According to the American Pharmaceutical Association, about 25 to 50 percent of prescription drugs contain at least one component derived from or modeled after a known plant."[1]

One of the persistent warnings emanating from certain health ideologues is "Watch out—herbs are harmful to your health!" When you compare the side effects of careless or indiscriminate usage of herbs or herbal supplements to those of the synthetic variety manufactured in chemical laboratories, the latter comes out as consistently more problematic.

You can always overdo a good thing, any good thing. However, to argue against the regular employment of nature's health–promoting plants is just plain foolish. If we would compare the deaths of people on multiple prescriptions in any year of the past decade to those of people mixing ginger, cinnamon, cayenne, basil, thyme, or any variety of roots and barks in moderate doses, the decision is an obvious wash; herbs and spices are safe in sensible quantities and have a much better historical record of safety and effectiveness than much of the synthetic and high–priced pills.

There are instances when a heroic effort is needed to save the body in emergencies and traumas, and this is the domain where modern medical technology excels. We must give credit where it is due. Antibiotics, for example, have been very effective in emergency situations. Unfortunately, we are now seeing the effects of the over-prescriptions of antibiotics, as bacteria are mutating in response to an inundation of medication.

Emergencies aside, for the other 99% of the time, we have nature to assist us in prevention or in a slow, safe, and lasting healing, assuming we cooperate with nature's design. There is much room for improvement in strengthening our immune system. The three major areas that have been regularly shown to bolster the immune system are regular exercise, stress management (which works in collaboration with a spiritual or ethical philosophy) and a quality diet, which in aboriginal cultures frequently includes plants as medicine.

Curiously, the same people who sensationally caution against the customary use of plants for medicinal benefits seem remarkably quiet when it comes to the bona fide statistical dangers of (1) hospitals being key harbors of numerous viral and bacterial pathogens, despite universal precautions and cleaning practices by the staff (you can catch more in a standard hospital than in most other public facilities); (2) the disturbingly high rate of iatrogenic deaths that occur every year;[2] (3) the excessive incidences of Adverse Drug Reactions (ADRs) that deteriorate your condition or even kill you. ADRs are the ill effects of drugs taken just as prescribed. According to a 1998 University of Toronto study, ADRs are the fourth leading cause of death in the U.S.;[3] (4) the prohibitive number of people seriously injured or killed by unnecessary or poorly performed surgeries.[4]

More information is being uncovered about drug dangers not being reported in the studies for the approval of some drugs. There appears to be a concerted effort by some drug companies to run experiments specifically designed to minimize the side effects of the drug being tested. This skews the data for a favorable result when the drug may have serious side effects. Clearly there is much room for improvement in the way regulatory bodies guard the health of the consumer who takes synthetic drugs.

No one can deny that there are problems on both sides of the healthcare aisle. Some representatives of the medical orthodoxy try to fortify the profile of their industry by thoughtlessly dismissing the effectiveness of any natural therapies. Conversely, in the entrepreneur-laden world of alternative therapies, there are many reasons to be skeptical of fantastic cure-all claims so commonly paraded. Not all things labeled "natural" or "organic" are, and not all products vilified as "dangerous" live up to their detractor's accusations. Hyperbole runs amuck in the holistic health business, to the same degree that subterfuge and strategic deception permeate the allopathic medical business. It is a murky swamp, whether conventional or complimentary therapies, but we have to navigate it and do our best.

If the tables were turned, in all fairness, applying the same candor of disclosure that the medical orthodoxy demands of legitimate natural therapies, there would be a mandatory disclaimer posted at the entrance to every major U.S. hospital—something akin to this:

> "Caution: usage of these premises without pre-visit homework on your part, thorough hand-washing while on the premises, *complete* submission to any of our doctor's notions, or haste in swallowing something for which the side effects or product safety record is still unknown may promote grave consequences. Remember to stop by our cafeteria for the jelly doughnuts and ninety-nine cent coffee."

Ranting put aside for the time being, we should not abandon the health benefits of plant medicines: roots, stalks, barks, leaves, and seeds. Hundreds of these plant-based properties have a very favorable track record, with the documented medicinal benefits of some herbs spanning over twenty centuries.

Herb versus Spice

An herb is derived from the leaf of a plant. A spice comes from the seed. Often, they both have health-promoting benefits. Coriander seed, for example, comes from the same plant whose leaves we enjoy as cilantro. Both have positive phytochemical effects upon the body.

Here are just a few headlines about plant medicine:

- **January 26, 2004**—The antibacterial, antifungal, antioxidant and anti-carcinogenic properties attributed to essential oils can be used as natural additives in a range of foods. New research into *basil* and *thyme* essential oils reveals their ability to curb *Shigella*, a harmful food-borne bacterium.[5]

- **2004**—One of the most talked about benefits of *cinnamon* relates to Type II diabetes. A study published in the *Journal of Diabetes Care* found that half a teaspoon of cinnamon a day significantly reduces blood sugar levels in people with Type II diabetes. It also reduces triglyceride, LDL cholesterol, and total cholesterol levels among this group.[6]

- **1999**—The IFT reports: Basil, rosemary, sage, mint, and other spices were found to be very active in an antitumorigenic activity test. This study indicates the potential antitumorigenic activities of spices. It may initialize extensive research on the healthy effect of spices.[7]

Hundreds of herbs and spices are used for their medicinal benefits.[8] Due to space limitations, the following will present the reader with twelve very popular herbs or spices with a brief explanation of their health-promoting advantages. Until you have gained more knowledge about the usage of each plant, it is not recommended that you mix too many herbs together, and please do not ingest herbs if you are pregnant without first consulting with a licensed herbalist, naturopathic practitioner, or other qualified expert in plant medicines.

There are formulas of plant mixtures already developed by experienced herbologists, nutraceutical researchers, and ethnobotanists, which anyone can make or acquire. In Chinese medicine, for instance, some of the herbal formulas used to treat disease have remained unchanged for over 800 years and are still effective. Get to know and appreciate the many benefits of nature's garden.

1. **Aloe Vera** (*Aloe barbadensis*)

This desert lily, or desert succulent, has a reputation as a healer. It is even mentioned in the Bible. Greek physicians used it for numerous ailments, from burns to constipation. Alexander the Great captured an entire island off the coast of Somalia for the sake of having this natural healing salve for his soldiers' wounds. The infamous Egyptian Queen, Cleopatra, is reported to have used aloe as an anti-aging ointment. The Egyptians appear to have employed aloe in their embalming recipes, which is perhaps one of the reasons that the New Testament mentions its use for the body of Jesus after he died.

Plant constituent used: the viscous gel inside the leaves

Therapeutic uses:

- Burns and skin abrasions. It speeds up the healing of new skin tissue and acts as a barrier against harmful bacteria.
- Bug bites, cuts, and minor skin irritations. It acts as a soothing topical anti-inflammatory.
- Internally taken for arthritis, heartburn and acid reflux, stomach ulcers, indigestion, and as a general detoxifier. You must ensure that you take specially prepared aloe for internal usage. Eating the gel straight from the plant is not recommended, as aloe contains very potent laxative chemicals called anthraquinones; excess dosage could cause abdominal cramps as well as diarrhea.
- Toxicity is very unlikely with internal usage of an ingestible-ready aloe formula, as your body will likely produce diarrhea to signal excess dosage. As with all plant medicines, be conservative in dosages until you get familiar with how your body responds.

2. **Angelica** (*Angelica archangelica*)

How could a medicinal herb named after the archangel Raphael be omitted from this list? As one legend goes, Raphael came to a monk during the European plague epidemic of the mid–seventeenth century and told him to employ this herb to protect the ailing citizenry. Since the bubonic plague is a bacterial disease, this may have been an excellent choice; research has shown angelica to have some anti–bacterial properties.

Another legend holds that this plant is named after the archangel Michael, the Great Defender, because it was known to bloom around Michael's feast day, May 8th. According to the herbal lore, Michael explained that this herb would ward off evil. The plant's species name, *archangelica*, honors Michael.

Angelica was a very popular medicinal herb in the European traditions, known to be suitable for a wide variety of ailments. It became very popular among doctors and garnered the reputation as the "immunity plant."

It is a well–liked herb in the Chinese medical tradition. As a group, the various species are known as *dong gui*, commonly referred to as "woman's ginseng."

Plant constituents used: root, leaf, seed. The most commonly utilized part is the root; the leaf and seed have a weaker effect.

Therapeutic uses:

- Topically, angelica tincture or balm increases circulation to the extremities and reduces inflammation (arthritis or rheumatism).

Internally:

- Never eat fresh angelica root. Drying the root eliminates the toxic level of the phytochemicals.
- Clears phlegm in the lungs due to bronchial problems. Angelica was widely used by the early American colonists for respiratory ailments. They were reportedly surprised to discover Native American healers using the dried root for the same purposes, especially for tuberculosis.
- Its antispasmodic property makes it ideal to relieve menstrual cramps; it has many uses specific for women in traditional Chinese medicine.

- Chinese angelica is shown by researchers to be beneficial for blood clotting. This could be good news for people with anemia but should be a caution for people with heart disease. If you are taking medicinal doses (usually in tinctures or pills) of any plant, you should be working with an herbalist.
- A tea made with angelica leaves is popular for indigestion.
- Some people enjoy a tea of the boiled root as an overall energy tonic.

3. **Arnica** (*Arnica montana*)

Another popular remedy in the European tradition, arnica is a very powerful herb. Goethe is noted to have drunk a tea from its leaves for his angina, but few herbalists today recommend internal use because of its proclivity for toxicity. It is much more commonly employed today as a topical remedy. If you have sore, achy muscles, a topical arnica gel or cream, or tincture, is highly recommended.

Plant constituents used: its yellow or orange flowers; commercially available in a cream or gel preparation for topical use.

Therapeutic uses:

- Very popular for bruises, inflammation (sprains and strains), myalgia.
- As a homeopathic internal remedy for shock, fright, or pain; it can even be given to animals for the same symptoms, with excellent results.

4. **Basil** (*Ocimum labiatae*)

Basil is derived from the Greek word for *king*. Many people think of basil as an essential ingredient of pesto or a good pasta sauce, but don't underestimate the power of this herb. There is an arcane mythology with basil: the Egyptians believed that the blossoms strewn over the tombs opened the gates of heaven; The Greek Eastern Orthodox church uses it upon its alters; the traditional mourners of India placed basil in the hands of their departed loved ones to guarantee a safe journey to the next world, as it was associated with the goddess Lakshmi, the wife of the god Vishnu (the preserver of life, who incarnates as Lord Krishna);

in the Jewish tradition, basil gives strength while fasting, even if just holding it in the hand or keeping it upon the body.

The reputation of basil did not always look this stellar. The Greeks and early Romans thought this herb was a symbol of aggression and madness. They believed that in order to grow genuinely fragrant basil leaves the farmer had to curse and yell at the seeds while they were being sown. Even today, a French saying reflects this old belief; "to sow basil," means to rant. Both the Greek doctor Dioscorides and the renowned Roman, Claudius Galen, physician to five Roman emperors, recommended against the internal use of basil. They were under the impression that this herb could cause the spontaneous presence of internal worms—or worse—madness. It took about 1,000 years for this legend to die and for basil to gain acceptance as a truly healing plant.

There are six general varieties of basil in the U.S., with dwarf basil and sweet basil being the most familiar. Basil is a relative of the mint family, and therefore all the medicinal uses of mint apply to basil, especially with regard to nausea, nervousness, headaches, and aromatherapy use.

Plant constituents used: the fragrant leaves, the flowering buds, essential oil.

Therapeutic uses:
- In aromatherapy, basil uplifts the spirits, counters depression, and eases nervousness.
- Inhaling the vapors of steamed fresh basil leaves helps to alleviate sinus congestion.
- Basil has a remarkable antibacterial and antimicrobial property. This makes the oil useful for cuts, abrasions, insect bites, and rashes. You can also apply freshly cut leaves to the skin. In India, basil oil has been successful in treating certain cases of acne; basil tincture has proven effective as well.
- A combination of basil, skullcap, rosemary, valerian, and chamomile makes a relaxing tea. This is a fragrant and tasty delight.
- Because of its antiseptic properties, you can take basil internally as a cleanser; it counteracts parasites, yeast, and minor bacteria. If you mix pulverized fresh basil leaves and fresh garlic with a little

extra virgin olive oil, you have a type of medicinal pesto, excellent for its antimicrobial and antibacterial properties. You can eat it or apply it topically to abrasions and stings.

- Some research has shown basil to enhance the immune system, increasing disease–fighting white blood cells by up to 20%.

5. **Black Cohosh** (*Cimicifuga racemosa*)

Traditionally, Native American tribes have used this popular root for various gynecological conditions. The word *cohosh* is Algonquian for "rough," reflective of this plant's gnarled roots. It was rediscovered in the mid 1990s after a German clinical trial showed its effectiveness in relieving hot flashes and menstrual pain. Many alternative practitioners recommend black cohosh (usually as an ingredient in a formula) for menopause, as it is popular as a natural alternative to estrogen replacement therapy (ERT).

Plant constituents used: root, tincture.

Therapeutic uses:

- Lessens the pain from menstrual cramps.
- Decreases the irritability associated with PMS.
- Prescribed for ailments associated with menopause. Although not widely accepted in American mainstream medicine, black cohosh is a popular remedy in Germany (as an ingredient in natural-based formulas) for its estrogenic action; it mimics the function of estrogen.
- Used in a formula to treat depression.
- Traditionally implemented for rheumatoid arthritis or osteoarthritis related to menopause. Some studies have shown it to contain anti–inflammatory potential.
- Helps alleviate skin irritations and inflammations by way of topical applications.

6. **Cayenne** (*Capiscum frutescens, Capiscum annum*)

Contrary to popular rumor, spicy foods do not give you ulcers. Excessive worrying about them giving you ulcers may be the real culprit. Spicy foods, and most of the peppers found in the Solanaceae family, appear to have a genuine medicinal effect on the body. Most peppers contain large amounts of vitamin C and magnesium, even more than citrus fruits do. Many North American indigenous tribes used a topical rub of cayenne to alleviate the pain and inflammation of arthritis and bursitis. The Mayans were known to mix cayenne with chocolate. It is a fantastic topical application for increasing circulation and creating vasodilation in blood capillaries. Hot peppers also stimulate neurotransmitter activity, producing a euphoric neuroendocrine effect and reducing symptoms of pain.

Plant constituents used: the fruit and the hottest part of the plant, the seeds.
Therapeutic uses:

- Cayenne and a little sesame oil mixed together and placed on the hands and feet, under gloves and socks, is a secret to some cold-weather sports enthusiasts for keeping joints warm.
- An old-fashioned arthritis remedy is cayenne, ginger powder, ashwaganda powder, and arjun powder mixed with olive oil and a little ghee. This is lightly heated and rubbed into the affected joints.
- Stomach ulcers—use a tincture of cayenne (Tabasco sauce, for example) in your food. Any hot pepper sauce would garner the same increase of circulation, aiding healing. Remarkably, it is actually good for your stomach. Worry and stress are the real problems to your stomach. If eating cayenne tincture is new for you, you may wish to start out with small amounts added to water to get used to the effects.
- Researchers have been learning more about the beneficial effects of the capsicum family of foods on blood fats since the late 1980s. Besides increasing circulation and reducing inflammation, cayenne appears to lower the LDL cholesterol in the blood, reducing the risk for blocked arteries. This is not the only thing that you would do for yourself if you have a family history of arteriosclerosis, but it could be part of an overall natural prevention program.
- Cold/flu natural remedy #21: Mix 12 ounces of spearmint tea with ½ teaspoon freshly pulverized ginger, 1 finely minced garlic

clove, 1 teaspoon fresh lemon juice, 1 teaspoon wild honey, and 2 pinches of cayenne pepper. Mix well, drink often, and kiss your bug good-bye.

7. **Dandelion** (*Taraxacum officinale*)

What to most people is just an annoying weed is, to the herbalist, a very important medicinal plant. This plant shares the same family as chicory, the Asteraceae family, and first appears in the European medical annals around the late fifteenth century.

The Native Americans have an established tradition of using dandelion for ailments ranging from skin conditions to anemia. It is naturally high in potassium, which helps the body regulate excess sodium for alleviating water retention.

The German immigrants of the 1700s, largely composed of Mennonites and Quakers, brought dandelion with them as a remedy for liver and kidney disorders. This would have been a smart strategy: one never knows what poisons will be inadvertently encountered in new territories, and the liver and kidneys are the two major detoxifiers of the body.

Very popular in traditional Chinese medicine and Indian ayurveda, this plant is prescribed for a wide variety of ailments from bronchitis to hepatitis. This plant's leaves have a continued use as a "spring cleaner," popular in salads and widely utilized as a general detoxifier.

Plant constituents used: leaf, flower, and root.

Therapeutic uses:

- Gout is considered a type of toxemia manifesting as arthritis. As a cleansing protocol, dandelion is often part of a detoxification formula for this and other similar pathologies.
- The Chinese version, Pu Gong Ying, has a wide variety of medicinal applications, from skin conditions to organ dysfunction.
- Used as a liver cleanser (often in concord with milk thistle seed) to detoxify the largest visceral organ after drug or alcohol excess and minor poisoning, it is also used to counteract the effects of early cirrhosis.
- This plant helps stimulate bile flow, possibly preventing gallstones. The German formula, Chol-Grandelat is a popular herbal

formula for gallbladder dysfunction; it contains dandelion, rhubarb, and milk thistle.
- Some naturopaths like to employ it in a formula for heart ailments accompanied by excess fluid retention.

8. **Evening Primrose** (*Oenothera biennis*)

This wildflower, native to America, was brought to Europe in the 1600s, eventually garnering the name "king's cure-all." Traditionally, indigenous people of the Americas have used it as a topical remedy for skin conditions, wounds, and bruises.

Most of the plants grown for commercial use today are for the seed oil, evening primrose oil (EPO). There have been an increasing number of studies concerning the effects of the essential fatty acids in the seed oil of evening primrose. EPO has proven effective for a number of conditions, as it contains the vital Omega-3 and Omega-6 essential fatty acids. As always, do not take this herb if you are pregnant without first consulting a knowledgeable health professional. Special note: people taking medication for seizures should not take EPO without a medical consultation.

Plant constituents used: seed oil, bark, stem, leaf, flower.

Therapeutic uses:
- The seed oil has many applications: reducing allergic symptoms, decreasing the effects of PMS syndrome and menopause, lowering excess LDL cholesterol and hypertension, and healing skin inflammation. Some preliminary studies with rheumatoid arthritis patients show some hopeful results in reducing symptoms of tenderness and pain in the joints. There have not been sufficient data showing a positive effect upon osteoarthritis yet, but based upon the traditional uses of this plant, it is a good candidate for inclusion in an herbal joint tonic blend.
- In parts of Europe it is common to use EPO topically for eczema.

9. **Garlic** (*Allium sativum*)

If herbologists were to create a list of most effective wonder herbs, garlic would likely be at the top of the list. This little bulb, first cultivated in central Asia, is lauded in the medical remedies of the ancient Greeks (see Hippocrates and Aristotle), Romans (see Celsus and Galen), Egyptians (mentioned in 22 formulas in the papyrus of 1550 BCE, the *Codex Ebers*, or *Ebers Papyrus*, which some believe to be the oldest medical text), the Chinese, and Arabic medical traditions, to name just a few. Ayurvedic medicine has a special place for its versatile properties, as do many traditional folk remedies. The renowned biologist Louis Pasteur discovered in 1858 that garlic could kill certain bacteria. Albert Schweitzer in the twentieth century employed garlic in Africa to treat amebic dysentery and cholera during his mission. Even in battle during WWI and WWII, when antibiotics were in short supply, garlic was used with great effectiveness to reduce septic infections and gangrene. The Russians used garlic so often, because of their high casualties reducing the antibiotic supply, that garlic earned the nickname "Russian penicillin." There are also indications that the ancient Roman army used garlic and wine to treat soldiers' wounds.

Garlic, along with its cousin the onion, has traditionally been known to cultivate fire in the body. This fire is equivalent to passion, which some societies channeled for warfare or labor. The early Buddhist and Christian monks of some sects considered garlic a forbidden food, as it would incite feelings of lust and physical passion, which are not exactly to a monk's advantage.

For its true medicinal benefits there has yet to be invented a successful substitute for fresh garlic; you must crush, chew, chop, or bruise fresh garlic in order to mix the medicinally inactive alliin with the potent antibiotic allicin; alliin by itself has no medicinal benefits. There is plenty of research validating garlic's medicinal effects; a few of the most notable follow.

Plant constituents used: the bulb, whole (for medicinal effect) or dried (for a more modest, culinary effect).

Therapeutic uses:

- Fresh garlic is antibacterial. You can rub it directly on cuts and abrasions (after cleaning) to reduce infection.
- Fresh garlic is antifungal. It is successful in treating athlete's foot (*Tinea pedis*) and vaginal yeast infections caused by *Candida albicans*.

- Reduces blood clotting and blood pressure, making it ideal for cardiovascular treatment and prevention. No other single plant-based medicine has more positive cardiovascular benefits than garlic.
- Reduces blood sugar levels in both humans and laboratory animals. This could be a very important dietary addition for diabetics.
- There are statistical links between a lower incidence of stomach and lung cancer and garlic consumption. Research is ongoing, studying garlic's anti-carcinogenic effects to see if it has wider applications; some researchers are very optimistic.[9]
- Boosts your immune system's activity, increasing the effectiveness of macrophages (the good cells that eat the toxins and viruses) and helper T-cells (which make you more resistant to disease).
- Lowers the "bad" cholesterol, the LDL, while raising the "good" type, the HDL.
- Reduces the risk of blood clots. The next time you have that 20-hour flight to Sydney, eat garlic before your flight. You can wear a little lemon oil and chew a few coffee beans to help counter the smell for your fellow passengers, and you may minimize the risk of deep vein thrombosis that occurs with long plane flights. Some researchers see garlic equal or superior to aspirin, much touted for its blood thinning capabilities.
- Garlic oil is good for indigestion. Indigestion recipe #276: in 6 ounces of ghee (clarified butter), heated slowly in a pan, add ½ teaspoon cinnamon, 1 teaspoon freshly pulverized ginger, ¼ teaspoon cardamom, ¼ teaspoon Jamaican allspice, a pinch of nutmeg, and a pinch of fresh lime zest. Stir in ½ teaspoon of garlic oil (usually fresh garlic infused in olive oil). Mix well and let cool to room temperature. Pour into a small sealable glass container and keep refrigerated. Add ¼ teaspoon to approximately 8 ounces of hot tea (preferably green tea) for indigestion.
- What to do about the smell? Some common remedies are chewing fennel seeds, coffee beans, or dark chocolate. Chocolate-cov-

ered coffee beans are offered in some restaurants with a garlic-heavy menu. If garlic is on your hands after cooking, try rubbing your fingers on a stainless steel utensil. The chemical reaction helps minimize the garlic smell on the skin.

10. **Nettle** (*Urtica dioica*)

Some 500 *Urtica* species grow throughout four continents. The alternate name is *stinging nettle* because the plant is composed of tiny spines that trigger a histamine release if they puncture the skin; yes, it stings. The name of the plant likely derives from an old European word for *needle*.

American strains of this plant have an innocuous effect compared to their tropical cousins. In other areas of the globe, a sting from a native nettle plant could produce burning sensations lasting for days (one Javanese species, *Urtica urentissima*, is described as having a sting that lasts a year!) and even symptoms that approximate lockjaw. Interestingly, if the leaves of American varieties dry out, the acids in the dried nettle leaves act as a natural antihistamine in the human body. There appear to be natural anti–asthmatic characteristics, as well. Naturopaths use nettle as an effective allergy and hay fever remedy.

Plant constituents used: leaf and root.

Therapeutic uses:

- Nettle tincture is used as a topical compress for skin problems and arthritis.
- Since it has anti–inflammatory properties, just about all pathologies ending with *itis* can be treated with nettles—arthritis, bursitis, tendonitis, and so on. Even hemorrhoids, a variety of inflammation, can be treated with a nettle cream.
- Nettle root is taken for heavy menstruation.
- Helps detoxify the body. Some herbs traditionally used for cleansing the tissues and blood include nettles, dandelion, milk thistle, and burdock root.
- Hay fever and allergies are treated with nettles.
- Recent research has shown great promise in treating patients with an enlarged prostate (in accord with saw palmetto berry) and in

preventing kidney stones. Nettle tea increases the flow and volume of urine, which assists in alleviating the symptoms.
- The ancient use of nettles for gout by urtication (purposefully sticking oneself with the plant's sharp spires) has been effective in a few studies.

11. **Sage** (*Salvia officinalis, Salvia sclarea, Salvia triloba*)
There are numerous varieties of this evergreen shrub throughout the world. Some estimates indicate over 500 species. Originally cultivated in the northern Mediterranean, this plant is used both as a spice and a medicine. Salvia finds its way to North America during the seventeenth century when folk healers employed it for many ailments, including intestinal worms, seasickness, and insomnia.

The Egyptians used salvia as a type of fertility elixir. The Greeks employed it for cleaning sores and wounds, stopping bleeding, and using it as a gargle for hoarseness and coughing. They also believed that it, along with rosemary, could enhance memory. The leaves worn on the side of the head in many Greek works of art are often salvia or rosemary. The ayurvedic tradition of India received salvia from the Greeks, and it became a popular addition to their herbal repertoire. From 1840 to 1900, sage was officially included in the United States Pharmacopoeia as a gargle for sore throats.[10]

From the Roman natural-medicine aficionado Pliny to France's illustrious king Charlemagne, many people used salvia, noted often for enhancing longevity.

The salvia strains with medicinal properties contain thujone, a highly antiseptic, fungistatic, and antimicrobial phytochemical. If taken in large doses, thujone is toxic. It is recommended that you do not ingest sage oil or tincture without professional guidance (pharmaceutical-grade salvia tincture is 1:10 leaf to ethanol).

Plant constituents used: leaves and essential oil.
Therapeutic uses:
- A traditional use of sage has been for sore throats. Make a tea from the dried leaves and add a little apple cider vinegar and honey. Then gargle. The astringent tannins in the salvia leaves

have an anti-inflammatory effect.

- Chewing on leaves has been used for inflamed gums or mouth sores. One could also rinse the mouth with a salvia infusion. The previously mentioned tannins act to reduce edema in delicate tissues.
- Sage tincture or infusion helps to minimize menstrual cramps.
- Some traditions refer to sage as a "woman's plant," as it is employed for alleviating menopausal symptoms, regulating periods, diminishing hot flashes, and alleviating depression.
- Sage tea is widely used to mitigate night sweats.
- Using sage to alleviate skin problems is popular.
- An emerging use for medicinal salvia is for lowering blood sugar levels in diabetics.
- More health product manufacturers are including sage in their deodorants. Sage is a natural candidate because of its antibacterial constituents, as bacteria are the cause of odors. Salysat, an antiperspirant made primarily of sage oil, is sold in Germany.

12. **Valerian** (*Valeriana officinalis*)

You cannot ignore the smell of valerian or the taste. Besides ranking high on the "worst smells" and "most bitter tasting" lists, this tall perennial is a valuable addition to your cupboard, especially if you need to relax (or know of someone who does). The medicinal benefits of valerian have been documented for hundreds of years. Researchers are still working on identifying valerian's active ingredients—we know what valerian does; we don't know exactly how it does it.

Plant constituents used: mostly the root.

Therapeutic uses:

- As a non-addictive mild tranquilizer, this plant's roots go to the head of the list, perhaps only rivaled by kava kava, which has a stronger narcotic effect and possible toxic consequences if taken in excess. Valerian is the natural sedative of choice by many because it has no known side effects.
- Currently, the German market is the largest for valerian root. The Europeans, in general, have a much more progressive approach

to natural therapies than the U.S.
- Some natural medicine cultures of South Africa, Central Asia, and Northern Europe have employed valerian for menstrual cramps and muscle spasms for centuries.
- Contemporary healers prescribe this root for anxiety, phobias, restlessness, and insomnia.
- It is common to find valerian in relaxation formulas that include skullcap, chamomile, lemon balm, and passion flower.

16

Cayce Case Studies

IN AN EFFORT TO EXAMINE SOME OF OUR NUTRITIONAL CONCEPTS in context with the Cayce readings, the following cases are noteworthy. These few examples have lessons that are relevant to a range of people trying to holistically understand their own health. Everyone has unique health concerns that can only be fully addressed by self–awareness and, if needed, collaboration with a knowledgeable health professional.

60-year-old female, readings for 618

Basic Problem:

This woman was having a difficult time with the cleansing processes of the body, physical as well as mental.

Pathology:

She had low blood pressure and poor arterial circulation, and an "engorgement" in the ascending portion of the large intestine first pro–duced by "an accumulation of phlegm." The reading explains further, "All of these are the effect, as it were, of the settlings of a cold germ that has produced—and does produce—this engorgement." The "cold germ" in this case is a type of virus that had proliferated because of excess mucus in the colon. It seems that she had a flu that settled in the lower small intestine and colon. Additionally, this woman had a prolapsed ascending colon because of the distention—the intestinal structure was essentially falling out of place.

She appeared to have "a tendency for the exercising of the mental forces ... in such measures and such ways as to make for disconcerting activity in the assimilations of the body." In other words, her mental choices were tending toward negative and anxious and this was affecting her digestion, which was affecting her overall health and disposition.

One of the energetic principles associated with the colon is the ability to "just let it go." Some people who harbor malice or acrimony for another have the emotional effects of their thoughts settle in the large intestine.

Mrs. 618 would likely have been a candidate for what we now call *irritable bowel syndrome* (IBS), with a prolapsed colon. IBS does not indicate a prolapsed colon; it just so happens that this particular person had both conditions.

Statistically, irritable bowel syndrome, chronic fatigue syndrome, migraines, and fibromyalgia all appear to operate together in some degree. Perhaps one day they will be ascertained as diverse aspects of the same central dysfunction. For now, many healthcare providers treat them as separate pathologies. There does appear to be a highly emotional component to each of these, coupled with various biochemical and metabolic imbalances; it is a bit of a chicken-and-egg scenario—emotions affecting body or vice-versa.

She also complained of vaginal pain, which she was informed was originating from the colonic distention putting pressure on her bladder and related organs.

Advice:

"Do not eat when excited. Do not eat because it is just time to eat. Eat when the appetite calls for it, and in most cases—as well as for this body—*what* the appetite calls for; but do not gormandize at any time." This is certainly wisdom for our own times: know when to say "enough" with food.

It was recommended that she stay away from meat and increase consumption of raw vegetables, likely for the fibrous benefit.

In a previous reading she was also asked to try the citrus fruit diet for two or three days, "to alkalize the whole system." Then she was to have a colonic (with baking soda succeeded by GlycoThymoline) after three days of the citrus diet. The colonics were to continue once a week for five to six weeks. After this cleansing phase, the Source suggested that the rebuilding phase should commence: "When these enemas have begun, change the diet to that which will be more substantial as to the rebuildings in the system."

Besides dietary advice, she was told to use an electric vibrator along the spine, especially the lower thoracic and lumbar vertebrae, and "Don't be overanxious, but keep quiet, even keel."

27-year-old female (first reading), readings for 2186

Basic problem:
This woman was having a difficult time in the building processes and chemical balances of the body.
Pathology:
She appeared to have a slight blood imbalance, a tendency towards anemia, and "with the lack of the structural bone and [sufficiency] of the calcium and supply of acids for the digestion in its proper relationships, [these] continue to prevent the body from body–building." She also had an endocrine inefficiency that appeared to result from her hyperactivity without sufficient repose. Because of a lack of vital energy in the blood, she had an "inflammation or weakness" in the nasal passages, head, and throat.
Advice:
The first direction the Source gave her was this: "We would be more careful as to the budgeting of the time. Take time for rest and recuperation. Take time for activities in which the exercising of the body–physical makes for resuscitation and not for detrimental conditions." This is a common problem today—not just in 1940 when this reading occurred. Many people don't exercise with the intention of rejuvenating their body as much as exhausting it. This is where the Asian movement arts have much to teach the West.

She was asked to refrain from carbonated beverages and alcoholic drinks, and instead to take "citrus fruit juices in quantities, regularly," and with a specific recommendation for a very alkalizing routine: "Drink at least a pint of orange juice, with the juice of half a lemon squeezed into same, each day; for periods of ten days—then leave off for a period of ten days, and then take again for another ten days, and so on."

She was given the formula for what we now call Inspirol for her nasopharyngeal difficulties, with the instructions to "inhale regularly of mornings upon arising, and of evenings when retiring. Inhale into one nostril, holding the other, then into the other side; also into the throat—letting the fumes go into the lungs—not swallowing the inhalant, but inhaling the fumes, see? Hold either side of the nostril as it is inhaled in the other nostril." This is the common manner for using Inspirol, which personal experience has proven to be very effective.

Miss 2186 returned for her second health reading about two years later. She had not improved because she still had a tendency towards being "overanxious," and she had not eliminated the "drosses" of the body. This is an old-fashioned way to say that she had a bit of a toxic backup in the tissues, which we discover is due to "poor digestions . . . and poor eliminations."

She was told in this reading that she had a tendency to be somewhat manic-depressive, as we would characterize it today. Also, she was to keep herself from being cold or damp, "prevent overacidity" in her diet, and establish "good eliminations."

Although the Source recommended in her health reading that she eat the fat of chicken, she was also to balance it by including some raw vegetables. In this reading, as in many others, portions are not advised according to percentages or specific amounts.

Besides recommending a calcium supplement (Calcios), raw milk with a digestive aid, and staying away from foods with vinegar and foods "that sour," she was advised to eat "a great deal of sea foods and chicken, and especially the bony pieces. Cook it like you would chicken and dumplings, but don't eat the dumplings—feed these to the dogs! Eat the bony pieces—and the greases of same are good for the body. Eat raw vegetables, and especially carrots. Have plenty of beets and beet tops in the diet."

Later, in her health reading of 1944 (2186-4) she was told, "There is still much to be desired by this body [because of an] inability of the assimilations." She was advised to take a digestive aid regularly in a glass of "fresh milk" and to exercise in the open to benefit from the "vital energies " of vitamins A and D "which will come from sunshine." Her central problem was identified as poor circulation and the incoordination of the "sympathetic and cerebrospinal systems."

In her first health reading she was told, in response to asking if she should change teaching jobs, " . . . if there is the giving out of self for HELPFULNESS, stay where you are!" Since none of us can escape the importance of understanding our spiritual imperatives, this reading counseled her: "there needs to be a better correlation with spiritual atmosphere, spiritual reactions within self. Be not only good,—be good FOR something!"

Miss 2186 remained teaching for 43 years and passed into spirit March 21, 1984, at age 71

Female, age unknown, readings for 5692

Basic problem:

This woman appeared to suffer from lack of both sufficient building reactions and cleansing in the digestive processes. She had a mixed form, in need of cleansing and building.

Pathology:

This woman had a number of physical imbalances including a dull, achy feeling through the lumbosacral area, sinus congestion, indigestion because of " [the] over amount of the hydrochloric forces," constipation, which "overtaxes . . . the rest of the viscera [organs]," and "some inflammation . . . experienced through the kidneys or the organs of the pelvis, overtaxed nervous strain."

She had intestinal lacerations that were utilizing extra white blood cells, essentially robbing her system of them. This could have predisposed her to a weakened immune system, causing her to be slower to heal.

Interestingly, in TCM kidney imbalances can manifest in lumbar pain and dysfunction; the associative emotional component is fearfulness or insecurity. The kidney energies could also be adversely affected by exposure to too cold of an environment, or by a lack or heating, warming foods.

Advice:

The Cayce Source recommended an interesting digestive tonic that included dried sage, gin and ambergris,[1] cane sugar, and cinnamon bark. This would be recommended a few other times and is the original formula for the clary sage water. Both sage and cinnamon have a natural anti-inflammation property, and energetically they are warming, stimulating herbs (although cinnamon is technically a spice, not an herb).

When asked if she was getting enough protein, the reply came as "Not sufficient. We are giving the diet as the body calls for it, see. The body has hindered itself by finding things disagreeing. With these properties as given, the body could digest 'nails' if they were taken, you see."

Perhaps one of the main concerns was that she was too finicky with food or just too emotionally unsteady. The advice given to her, which echoes throughout ancient healing traditions, is "Control the body with the mind forces."

Miss 5692 did not follow the directions specifically as recommended, and after two sessions, about 2½ months apart, she discontinued involvement with the readings.

6-year-old female, readings for 4281

She received 17 readings total, from 1923 to 1928.

Basic Problem:

This child appeared to suffer from the inability to process sugars and an intestinal imbalance. The dilemma here was the balance between building functions needed for tissue production and cleansing processes needed to rectify a pancreas digestive inefficiency, especially with the sensitivities of a young child.

Pathology:

The child was diagnosed with celiac disease, which is an intestinal malabsorption syndrome commonly manifesting diarrhea and, often, calcium insufficiency. It is common for this pathology to produce some kind of malnutrition because of the absorption difficulties. Today we understand celiac disease much better in relationship to nutrition. Much of what we know about blood and metabolic typing and purine consumption addresses the effects of this pathology.

There also appeared to be a nerve impingement to some degree of the thoracic vertebrae 7–10, which the reading recommends having rectified. Nerve supply to the pancreas and duodenum (part of the small intestine) was also mentioned as needing "stimulation."

Advice:

Milk was recommended "in small quantities, without heating." The source of the milk was important, according to the reading; the advice suggested that "care should be given to the supply from which this milk is obtained, and had best be from that source where principally dry food is given, for this supply with the new vegetation would be detrimental. [It] Will be beneficial farther along in season." Since this reading was given in March, we can assume that she was taking milk from cows eating late winter and early spring plants. This may have provided insufficient chlorophyll in the plant for appealing milk production. The later seasonal plants of spring would have been richer in chlorophyll and produced better–quality milk. This was Dr. Weston A. Price's nutritional anthem: to eat butter from cows who have fresh–growing, chlorophyll–rich grasses in the spring. The quality of fats, he asserted, are vastly superior and crucial to excellent somatic development.

In a previous reading for this child the advice was to take "Bulgarian buttermilk . . . seasoned with salt and pepper." This was another rich fuel and body–building source for the child. Perhaps the seasoning mitigated the natural sour taste, making it more palatable for the little girl.

The next bit of advice warned against using any kind of table sugar for this child. "Not too much sugar, even of the beet sugar, but do not use raw cane sugar in any manner. Saccharin would be better even than the beet sugar." Saccharin was invented in the late 1800s and was recommended by the Cayce Source numerous times as a feasible sugar substitute in moderation. Numerous researchers have refuted the experiments of the 1960s and 1970s touting Saccharin as carcinogenic. The problem is that once a product has been labeled as dangerous in the eye of the public, it is branded for life, despite the facts. These days, no one runs news stories warning you of the destruction your pancreas cells will undergo with habitual consumption of refined cane sugar. You will hear that adult–onset diabetes is expanding amongst the population at a phenomenal rate but not that your refined sugar addiction is slowly killing you. And let's be frank: Even if someone did tell a person this, would he listen?

Another recommendation advises the following: "Whole pure wheat, rolled, and this made in gruel would be excellent for [the] system." The readings state that she needed more salivary activity to bolster her digestion and that eating whole grains would certainly help that, as the enzymes produced in the saliva occur naturally to break down the starches.

No meat was to be taken by this little girl but the juices of "clean beef [kosher?]." The Source also recommended, "Do not give meats, save fish or wild fowl. No tame fowl." Beef juice is a common recommendation in the readings as a good body–building food. The amino acids in organic beef broth (not the dehydrated, processed version) are excellent for gaining strength in the body.

Diet and spinal adjustments were a continual recommendation in this young girl's 17 readings. In her last reading she was given the Inspirol recipe for a cough and told that she was progressing very well and to keep away from sweets. When asked how to reduce her sweet craving, the common sense advise was "to keep them away from the body." We could call this the "out of sight, out of mouth" approach.

She was healthy enough to start public school for the first time in 1928.

48-year-old female, readings for 255

Basic Problem:
This is a good example of the yin–yang principle and how it func-

tions in the body. Building processes, a yang function, needs to be balanced with cleansing processes of the body, a yin function. Balance is the key, as the readings emphasize repeatedly, in rest and work, thinking and action, cleansing and building. This woman decided to get a physical reading for herself while her daughter was being treated in the Cayce hospital, and she received a valuable prompting to get her act together.

Pathology:

Her first reading dealt with her only complaint: constipation. But the Cayce source cautioned her that although this seemed like a trivial complaint, it could manifest as a greater problem later: "The body should be warned; for while the conditions at the present do not cause such distress, but rather inconveniences, yet were the conditions to be allowed to remain, the conditions *builded in* the system must eventually *affect* the system in a manner as would be hard to combat."

Important Lesson Number One from this reading: Don't interpret chronic constipation as a minor situation. Toxic back up in the colon quickly affects your entire system and needs to be promptly addressed with natural means.

She also had a problem with the quality of her hemoglobin and blood coagulation, likely from a poor diet and excess inactivity and not from any genetic factors.

Advice:

Osteopathic adjustments were to be made along the spine, especially in the lower lumbar and sacral–coccygeal nerve plexuses; it appeared that her tailbone was out of place, which was causing both physical and emotional "nervousness and uneasiness." She is informed in her sixth reading that she has muscular forces too strong in some directions and too weak in others that contribute to this skeletal misalignment—a yin-yang imbalance.

Her constipation was also producing early signs of liver and colon trouble, often signs of chronic stress. The normal peristalsis of the gastrointestinal tract was impeded by her inability to regularly relax. This is a common occurrence with people who are "stuck" in sympathetic fight-or-flight responses. Your body needs permission to relax and feel safe in order for digestion to function favorably. The yang condition of the body, when you prepare it for combative engagement or innate escape by a given mental decision, needs to be balanced by the yin phase of rest-and-repose, also a mental decision.

The yin function of being relaxed, which a person needs to rejuvenate the body, can be taken too far, as well; you can harm the body just as much by inactivity as by hyperactivity. The Cayce source told her, "the body *poisons* self by the sedentary conditions as accumulate there [in the intestines]." Important Lesson Number Two from this reading: Both exercise and appropriate rest are medicine for your body.

The next important lesson, Number Three, follows closely with the advice: It is not how much you weigh as much as how healthy you are with your weight. Trying to create a single height-to-weight index that will apply equally to such a vastly diverse ethnic population as the one in America can be enormously misleading: "More consideration should be given to health, than to [what] . . . the weight is . . . average or normal." In other words, it is not necessarily quantity that is the main problem, but quality. Some people have a genetic propensity to be big boned, as they say, but they are not consequentially unhealthy just because they fall outside of the theoretical height-to-weight index. As a matter of fact, many social advocates have observed how ethnocentric these indices can be, working to the disadvantage of many people of African, Mesoamerican, and Polynesian heritages, to name just a few. If the tables were turned, a thin Caucasian might be considered emphatically emaciated in another culture and be socially ostracized because of it.

When you exercise and replace fat cells with muscle cells, since muscle weighs more than fat, you will weigh more, even though you are healthier. Don't go just by weight but by how you feel.

In her follow-up reading two months later (reading 255-2), the woman is advised that the same conditions are present and that her eliminations need to be regulated; just as toxins are thrown off by the lungs and kidneys (excess carbon), so too with the colon.

In her third reading about three weeks later, she received the real medicine: "While there are conditions as disturb the body, these—as we find—have more to do with the mental attitude than with physical conditions." It is time to get your mental house in order, sister, to paraphrase the Buddha.

Just to illustrate how we really do not listen to what people say, right after being told that her mental choices were affecting her physical health, does she inquire specifically about that? No. She asks about saccharin. The info we get on saccharin is interesting, but her opportunity for uncovering the roots of her psycho-emotional distress are being squandered by not paying attention to what the Cayce source was advising. This is a very common occurrence in the readings. And to be fair, this was a highly unusual way to get assistance at a time when it likely appeared as a novelty of sorts. It is also basic human nature. We have not culturally evolved far past the same antiquated view today. Viewing the readings in retrospect, you often find yourself asking "Why didn't they just ask *why* more?"

The point the Source makes about saccharin is an intriguing one: "[Saccharin] should be good for the body, for it supplies more of the carbons in the system, and is the active principle of sweet that forms the basis of the active forces in the gastric juices . . . or those of proper fermentation in the system, and it is better than those that come of cane, corn, or of others, save the conditions wherein the sweets from *beet* are better than saccharin." Beet sugar was preferred as a sweetener, but next in preference for this person was saccharin.

We secondly receive interesting information about iron-rich foods. The best, according to this reading, are oranges found in the southern states, especially the Rio Grande Valley; next are the citrus fruits located in Florida; lastly, the citrus of California. Next, "spinach . . . cabbage . . . turnips . . . salsify . . . radish, and of such natures. These add to the system. In the fruits, and for *this* body—well that pears be eaten . . . [also] some [varieties] of apples . . . "

She was also given valuable advice for building nerve tissue through dietary means: " . . . [Eat] those of the celery, radish, those of the *green* vegetables, [and same] in tomatoes. Those of the active forces in these are the nerve building, with those of the *juices*—but not the flesh—of animal." This would be in keeping with yogic advice that green foods are digestively cleansing and energetically building foods. According to this same philosophy, animal proteins have too much animal–passion vibration for a person who is already a nervous wreck. Advice for most anyone: vegetarian diets can be utilized as part of an inner cleanse—mental and physical—even if you choose not to remain on it as a regular habit. Try it; you'll like it—at least your body will.

In case we get too sanctimonious in our nutritive certainty, the sixth reading for Mrs. 255 holds a bit of cold water for our closely held *ism:* "To say that *any* diet that adds proper forces to the body for blood, muscle and nerve building, is in error, is to cut self off—even as to say, 'This I may do, this I may *not* do', see?" So even if you are a militant card-carrying vegan, you may greatly benefit at times of certain duress from meat broths or dairy. And those 20–ounce steak eaters would likely do their bodies a valuable service by having periodic vegetarian cleanses. Whatever our dietary viewpoint, let us not cling so tightly to one vantage as embrace many possibilities.

The diet recommended for her in this reading was essentially fruits only for breakfast, vegetables only for lunch (the ones given to her previously in the reading), and nuts (we can logically add seeds and legumes) in the evening. She was in need of digestive and eliminative efficiency, which proper food combining and simplification help attain.

This reading finishes with a classic bumper sticker quote: "Expect something, and something will happen! Do not expect anything, and most anything *may* happen!" She still needed to address her mental attitudes regarding health and healing, as do we all.

In reading number 7, the health of Mrs. 255 starts to take a turn for the worse about one year after her initial physical reading. This, we are told by the Cayce source, is because of "a *combination* of effects, or affectations for the system. These are *partially* astrological, partly from the change in the blood conditions—in the period or portion of the year—partially from those effects of conditions in the system as related to the *digestive* system, especially as to the gall ducts and the eliminations."

Some recommendations for her: castor oil packs over the liver; drinking alternating servings of cinnamon water and lime water; osteopathic adjustments (which would have implied massage therapy, as well); a salt and soda enema, with the addition of GlycoThymoline; a diet of citrus and crackers.

In the subsequent reading she was advised to take regular amounts of pure olive oil to "Grease self well throughout." This advice is reiterated in the next reading, number 9: "*nothing* is much better than the olive oil as a food for the intestinal system."

In reading number 10, her diet was modified to include citrus and stewed fruits in the morning, green salads in the afternoons, with the explicit recommendation that follows:

> "Keep the mental attitudes properly in their seasons, especially when supplying food for the resuscitating of the system, and seeing—as it is taken—that as *is* to be accomplished *by* that taken, *knowing* what each property is to supply to the system, and see it being accomplished."
>
> This would be counsel to eat mindfully, having imaginative mental forces assist with the body's healing.
>
> Evening meals could be the heaviest of the three, including cooked vegetables (especially the ones previously suggested) and seafood.

After this reading, she did not pursue much in terms of physical readings, but instead she sought to understand her life readings in a deeper manner. The notes tell us that she started getting her mental and spiritual life together, especially after the nervous breakdown of her husband. She is noted as incorporating many of the physical recommendations throughout the years, and these assisted her in being more physically active. Her spiritual life became more intensified, and she appears to have made substantial development.

She was active and in good health until a few months before her death, on October 28, 1967.

Appendix

Questions and Answers

MOST PEOPLE READ A BOOK LIKE THIS TO ANSWER A BASIC QUES-
tion: what should I eat? As I have tried to convey in the previous chapters, this is a complex question with a number of possibilities. Anyone
who tells you otherwise is being less than honest.

This truth withstanding, there are some generalizations that can be
applied, more or less, to most everyone. So, to get to the heart of the
matter, I will present actual questions (or slightly modified versions)
from friends, acquaintances, and students and answer them with the
best information I have at the present. This is not meant to represent a
standardized view of nutrition, as there really is not one, and if there
were, it would likely be obsolete by the time it was reliable. This is my
viewpoint on nutrition, based on years of research, study, and trial-
and-error.

1. What foods are known to fight disease?

The foods that would fit into the "disease fighting" category most
neatly are ones considered antioxidant-rich foods. Of course, we cannot
take an oversimplified view of this and expect nutrition to be a sole
cure-all. Good health requires a holistic approach, being aware of our
choices on multiple levels. However, thinking of food as medicine, we
would hardly find a better candidate in the vegetable group than dark
leafy-greens (DLGs).

DLGs consist of spinach, kale, chard, asparagus, green peppers, Brussels sprouts, broccoli, and most other leafy green edible plants. There is ample research on the benefits of these chlorophyll–loaded foods and the many health advantages they contain. If you want to increase your dietary intake of just one food, make it dark leafy–greens. You may want to increase your intake of more than just one food as well as eliminate the detrimental foods in order to maximize vitality.

In the larger context of antioxidant foods, the following all qualify as antioxidants and have confirmed benefits, assuming there are no food allergies:

• The carotenoid family, especially beta carotene foods—most all foods rich in colors red, orange, and yellow: carrots, sweet potatoes, red and yellow peppers, apricots, mangoes, and cantaloupe.

• Foods high in vitamin E: most of the DLGs, nuts and nut butters, seeds, whole grains, legumes, olive oil, and wheat germ.

• The vitamin–C laden foods: citrus fruits, tropical fruits, berries, cherries, peppers (green, red, yellow), tomatoes (vine–ripened), and DLGs. Peppers and berries have a higher vitamin C content then even citrus. Keep in mind that if you cook vitamin C foods this depletes the vitamin potential. To get the most from these foods eat them raw.

2. I have been told I need to increase my calcium intake to stop the osteoporosis that has recently come on in the last few years. What calcium–rich foods should I eat and what are the best calcium supplements?

Osteoporosis is a condition where the biochemical process that builds bone cells with calcium is being undermined by the cells that tear-down calcium, resulting in a perpetual net loss of the most abundant mineral in the body. To simply eat more calcium–rich foods is not the sole answer to this problem but could be part of a complex of helpful actions.

The first thing that you need to do is work with a healthcare practitioner who specializes in treating bone pathologies or who has a reputation for successfully treating osteoporosis. You need to get to the root cause of *why* you are losing bone mass, as there are numerous and diverse reasons. Once the "why" is established, the next step is determining the correct type of calcium supplement, as not all calcium prod-ucts on the market are the same, as well as the foods and activities to avoid. One common set of recommendations is to completely forsake all soft drinks, lower your salt intake, reduce or eliminate all alcohol consumption, exercise more, and switch to decaffeinated beverages.

As far as supplements are concerned, some people thrive on calcium citrate while others do well on coral calcium or other versions. How you metabolize nutrients will then determine what calcium-rich foods are most indicated for you personally.

With that qualification, here are some of the most common sources of dietary calcium:

• All dairy products. The milk of mammals is a very nutritious sub-stance in its natural unadulterated form. It is nature's perfect food for growing babies. Since milk is rich in calcium, phosphorus, and fats, and other valuable building materials for the body, dairy will naturally con-tain the same. Remember, *not all milk is equal*. There are considerations to recall regarding the quality of the milk: is rBST added? Is the milk cer-tified organic? Is the milk pasteurized? (This means heating it up in order to kill harmful bacteria. In doing so, the beneficial enzymes that help digest the milk are also destroyed.) Usually, adults can handle dairy in a fermented form (as they do all over the world with no conse-quences). This would include cheese, yogurt, cottage cheese, kefir, and the like. The rawer and fresher the milk, the better. Keep in mind that these are usually high in fat as well so you would want your activity level to be appropriate for a higher fat intake.

• Meats (fish and fowl are fine choices) are naturally high in cal-cium because the muscles are a natural storehouse of calcium; you need adequate calcium availability for contracting muscle tissue, which is located in the muscle and connective tissues. Boiling animal bones for a stew is an old-fashioned yet effective way to obtain dietary calcium. Once again, ensure that the animal has been well-raised and is chemi-cal-free.

• These are some popular vegetable-based sources of calcium: col-lard greens, parsley, and most of the DLGs (spinach, kale, mustard greens, etc.). Also, dried beans, (especially black, navy, adzuki, and mung beans), almonds (the highest of all nuts), and soybeans have a superior calcium content.

3. Exactly how important is it to avoid certain food combinations?

Generally speaking, the weaker your immune system or the more digestive problems you have the more you should focus on good food combining. There are some people, generally most healthy people under age 30, who can eat just about any outlandish combination of foods and recover unjeopardized. Once you start having health problems, approach middle age, or have a cold/flu bug, it is wise to pay attention to the rules of food combining. It is also smart to practice the rules of food combining if you have any gastrointestinal pathologies: Irritable Bowel Syndrome [IBS], diverticulitis, colitis, acid reflux syndrome, and chronic constipation are some of the most common troubles.

Many of the people Edgar Cayce counseled in the health readings received recommendations for food combining. The majority of people coming for health readings were already in dire straits health-wise and food combining was a sensible recommendation to enhance the functioning of their distressed immune system. Under normal circumstances the GI tract is quite robust and can adapt to many nutrient combinations, assuming the proportions are in moderate amounts and the person is basically in good health.

Some people find that certain food combinations provide exceptional results. Even with good health abounding there are food combinations that can be exceptionally advantageous for you; you have to experiment and see what works best. A couple of the most egregious combinations that the Cayce health readings recommended against are: mixing citrus and dairy at any time; mixing citrus and cereals; adding cream to coffee; frying foods, especially with "hog fats"; simple sugars with starches; simple sugars and meats.

4. Are there foods that promote longevity?

What I understand that question to ask is, "Can I eat something and live longer as a result?" The answer in brief is: probably not. None of us is going to get out of this incarnation alive. The focus of good nutrition and holistic living is not in just trying to extend the years of life but rather the life in the years. Every month, it seems, another study appears in the mainstream touting the virtues of numerous habits that researchers assume are adding to longevity in some demographic: eating breakfast is better than skipping it, drinking alcohol is better than not, meat eaters versus the vegans, and the list keeps growing. There are compelling arguments to be made on either side of these issues, and each side has their statistics, so perhaps determining one's lifespan is much more complicated than simply what one eats. If there is one dietary habit you can incorporate, and this is no guarantee of longevity as much as vitality, it is eating more fresh fruits and vegetables; the antioxidant foods that have been previously mentioned.

There are five other lifestyle habits you can cultivate to "stack the deck" in your favor:

1. **Keep a positive attitude,** as it all comes down to perspective. Taking care of your mental health should be a high priority. Some of the healthiest elders I have known keep the virtues of laughter as their close companion. Even if you have to go younger than you want (which is probably most of us) wouldn't it be best to go out laughing?

2. **Companionship** is good for your health, even with pets. Across the research spectrum it seems that people who are married, have pets, or who live in community (like monastics) appear to have a longer life span. It may be as simple as doing something that keeps you connected to your heart, which loved ones, pets, and a shared religious devotion all facilitate.

3. Smoking cigarettes is a killer, plain and simple. If you want a few more years, **drop the nicotine habit.** It is true that native Americans have a long tradition of smoking tobacco leaves, and they have chiefs who lived to be over 100. This is not the same as smoking modern cigarettes, which are far removed in form from pure tobacco leaves.

4. **Stay active.** A sedentary life is much more problematic to your health than an active one. Find excuses to walk more, swim, or hike in the beauty of nature. Get out and get involved in service and community events. Your body was made to move—put it to good use.

5. **Keep learning, keep growing.** Your mind needs exercise just like your body. Playing games that make you think, like chess or checkers, is good medicine for your mind. This could be applicable to cards, puzzles, and a host of board games. Even doing the daily crossword puzzle in the newspaper is a good start. Whatever it is, find something that works for you that you can do regularly to keep your mind sharp. As the old adage goes, and it is true: if you don't use it (or you misuse it), you lose it.

5. I hear that water supplies are contaminated by many chemicals. Is the tap water safe to drink?

The water supply in the U.S. is one of the safest and most tested in the world. Some people are under the assumption that all bottled water is superior to all tap water. According to the Natural Resources Defense Council's report of March 1999, between 20% to 40% of the bottled water you pay between 90¢ to $2.50 per gallon (or more) for comes from the tap. This report also reveals the disturbing fact that safety standards for bottled water are much lower than municipal tap water in most cities. There are state certified laboratories you can contact through the EPA's Safe Drinking Water Hotline at 800–426–4791.

You can also buy water filters to assist in purifying your tap water supply. The most expensive ones are not always the best value. As of January 2005, the average price for an effective water filter is between $120 and $160. Replacement cartridges for 500 gallon capacity units range from $45 to $55. There are various purification technologies from ultraviolet light to multi–chamber screen filtering but distillation, carbon filtering and reverse osmosis water filtration are the most common on the market.

Distillation is steam that is captured, condensed, and returned to a liquid. It has most all of the trace minerals removed from it. If you drink distilled water you should add tiny amounts of a liquid trace mineral supplement. Distillation systems are often costly, take up considerable space, and use quite a large amount of electricity. It also may not remove all harmful chemicals and pathogens, especially if you have water from a well.

Reverse osmosis is used by most of the commercial water bottling facilities. This technology uses a specialized micro-filter that traps particles too big to pass through a selective membrane, which includes heavy metals, lead, asbestos, and other dissolved chemicals. This process also removes minerals from the water. Often, reverse osmosis systems are used in conjunction with carbon filtering, also known as carbon absorption. The two primary types of carbon filtering are granular activated carbon and solid block carbon; both appear to work with equally effectiveness. The carbon acts as an extra filtration device to the reverse osmosis membrane, removing the unpleasant taste of chlorine and other chemicals.

Whatever choice you make with water filters, do your homework first. They all have convincing arguments why their system is the best creation, which is the nature of sales. One site that may be useful is: www.waterfiltercomprisons.net/Waterfilter_Comparisons.dfm.

The bottom line is that, so far, our water system is safe. You have to be more concerned about bottled water, especially if the water is being stored in hot locations as there may be some leaching of the plastic compounds into the water. You will know this usually by the strongly unpleasant taste of the water, kind of a chemical aftertaste.

6. What can I find in my grocery store that is healthy? It seems like everything is made with hydrogenated oils and high-fructose corn syrup.

It is difficult once you start reading labels and the realization, "Wow, I never knew commercial lasagna was made with so much sugar" dawns on you. One choice is to find a natural grocer in your area and support them, or you could talk with the manager of the local Food Mart and ask if they can special order some items for you. Next, there are online resources that will ship natural food products to you directly. Lastly, when in doubt, learn how to make it yourself with good, healthy ingredients.

7. How do we vegetarians get enough protein?

Thank goodness that whole grains and legumes mixed together act as a kind of complete protein. They have all the essential amino acids needed by the body. This is why rice is such a staple in many parts of the world. In some places, meats are such a valuable food (because there is not a surplus) that they are eaten only on special occasions. The rest of the year people live on rice, millet, quinoa, amaranth, barley, wheat, spelt, etc. If you add a variety of beans and lentils to the mix you are on the right road. Many of these cultures also incorporate a small amount of dairy, which is a protein-rich.

If you are a vegan, it is far more challenging, since animal products contain minerals and fats that our body needs. You may not be able to build muscle mass as a vegan but you can have vitality and good health with a wide variety of plant-based foods.

8. Is there a single resource I can rely on to make weekly menus? What is a good format to follow?

Unfortunately, (or fortunately, depending on how you look at it) there is not a singular source for any of this. Many people will tell you they have *the* answer for all your dietary needs but the truth is, only you can figure out what works for you. If you apply the basic concepts we have covered and keep your eyes and ears open for other helpful bits of information you will have all you need. Some basic common sense rules can help everyone if they actually put it into practice:

• Do not eat your biggest meals in the evening, especially if you are trying to lose weight.

• Do not over eat at any meal. You should learn to abide by the "enough is enough" maxim.

• If you are protein dominant in your metabolic constitution make sure that you have protein for breakfast, even if just a small amount.

• If you are trying to lose weight, do not snack on convenience foods. This would include basically anything you would find in a standard vending machine. Instead, eat fruits and vegetables as a snack—the more, the merrier. Instead of fried potatoes and pastries try: celery and organic peanut butter, apple and almond butter, sliced carrots, jicama and radishes wrapped in lettuce leaves, orange and tangerine wedges with bamboo shoots (you skewer them together with toothpicks), polenta with dried cranberries and cinnamon (sweetened with a little stevia powder), sliced celery root dipped in a balsamic vinegar and olive oil mix. There are countless other creative combinations you can try.

9. How important is "how" I eat, and what are some important guidelines to follow?

This is a very interesting question and one that could be a book in itself. To get the most from your foods you should coordinate your thoughts with your body. To eat prayerfully transforms the essential vibration of the food as it enters your body. The reverse of this can also happen where you eat good, well-made food but in a rushed, anxious, or angry manner and your digestive system becomes disrupted in the process.

This question is bigger than foods though. How you live your life, the journey along the way, is the real focus and not merely a certain destination. Many people rush through their lives trampling over people and nature looking for that ever-evasive "there" over there, one that they never find. Many people also are never aware of what they are eating, and if their body really wants it—they are all the same manifestation of unmindful living. If you start to work on being more mindful, expanding your internal awareness, how you eat will naturally change for the better.

Endnotes

Introduction

i. http://www.harrisinteractive.com/harris_poll/index.asp?PID=288
ii. According to U.S. Census Bureau—http://www.census.gov/main/www/popclock.html
iii. http://www.cdc.gov/nccdphp/factsheets/death_causes2000.htm
iv. http://www.cdc.gov/nccdphp/burdenbook2002/index.htm

Chapter One

1. *Present Moment, Wonderful Moment*; Thich Nhat Hanh, Parallax Press, Berkeley, Ca. 1990
2. Paraphrased from Psalm 111:5
3. Paramahansa Yogananda, *God Talks with Arjuna, The Bhagavad Gita*; Self-Realization Fellowship, Los Angeles, Ca. 1995. Page 996
4. *Dhammapada, The Sayings of the Buddha*; rendered by Thomas Byrom, Shambala, Boston, MA. 1993
5. *Dhammapada, The Sayings of the Buddha*, ibid.
6. Psalm 46:10

Chapter Two

1. Soma is the Greek root word meaning body. It is used in the context of somatic or, as many people have become familiar with it, psychosomatic (mind–body).
2. Peristalsis is the involuntary muscular contraction of the gastrointestinal tract that moves foods in a wave-like motion, from the esophagus to the rectum.
3. Self-Realization Fellowship, Los Angeles, Ca. © 1995
4. Fascia shares the same Latin root with the word fascist; Latin—fascio, "to band or bundle [together.]" Webster's, Random House, New York, NY. 1996
5. According to Gary Null Ph.D, there are 783,936 fatalities annually form iatrogenic reactions. He and others believe that this number is actually under-reported, with the actual statistic being considerably higher. http://www.garynull.com/documents/iatrogenic/deathbymedicine/DeathByMedicine3.htm
6. You can consult a free web site for more information, like this one created by the University Medical Center of Dijon, France: www.pneumotox.com. As always, do your homework on what drugs your doctor(s) prescribe for you; know the side effects, health risks, and track record of the drug in advance of taking the chemical.

Chapter Three

1. A sugar is called a saccharide in the body. A simple sugar is a monosaccharide (one sugar), and a long chain of sugars is called a polysaccharide, which is the same as a complex carbohydrate, a.k.a. a starch. Yes, it is common in anatomy sciences for one structure to have multiple names.
2. There are various statistics on this, as with other anatomical facts. Here are just a few examples:
    "18 to 20 feet:" Avraham, Regina. *The Digestive System.* Chelsea House, 2000: 52.
    "About 23 feet:" "Intestine." Encyclopedia Americana. Danbury, CT: Grolier, 1999: 323.
    "About 7 meters long:" *Gray's Anatomy* online, http://www.bartleby.com/107/248.html

Chapter Four

1. You can read about this from many authors. Here are just a few:
   1. *Eat Fat, Lose Weight: How the Right Fats Can Make You Thin for Life* Keats—1999; ISBN # 0-87983-966-X by Ann Louise Gittleman, MS., C.N.S.
   2. *Know Your Fats: The Complete Primer for Understanding the Nutrition of Fats, Oils and Cholesterol* by Mary G. Enig, Ph.D. ISBN# 0967812607
2. A recommended website for updates and information regarding fish supplies is the Monterey Bay Aquarium: http://www.mbayaq.org/cr/seafoodwatch.asp
3. "I talked about the dangers of white flour and sugar over 50 years ago, and people thought I was some kind of fool. Now it's every doctor: 'salt, white flour, sugar—killers, killers, killers'," he said, punching his couch for emphasis. "It's exciting what's happening. This is going to be the salvation of America; you watch and see. The incidences of drugs, alcoholism and crime on our streets will decrease in the next few years. Young people turn to drugs from eating too much sugar and refined, dead foods, and the lack of exercise. "How do you think kids get started on this deadly drug habit? It all starts with excessive consumption of white sugar, candy, soft drinks, etc. When you use too much sugar it destroys the B-complex vitamins, you can't make wise decisions, your energy's down and you're apprehensive and doubtful about your life. These are the hard facts. If you stop eating white sugar products and get on live, organic, natural foods, you will feel better immediately! Look at me; if Dr. Bragg hadn't changed my life at 15, I would have been dead at 17."

Jack Lalanne

From: http://www.bragg.com/company/about_jack.html

4. What should be eliminated are refined starches of all varieties.
5. ICM stands for Intestinal Clogging Material, an acronym that I devised years ago—all foodstuffs that are artificially modified.
6. Peristalsis is the involuntary muscular contraction of the gastrointestinal tract that moves foods in a wave-like motion, from the esophagus to the rectum.

Chapter Five

1. For more information see: *Eat Right For Your Blood Type*, Dr. D'Adamo, Peter J., Putnam; New York, NY. 1996.
2. Gen. 4:10; *The Amplified Bible*, Zondervan Publishing, Grand Rapids, MI. 1987
3. *Red Gold, The Epic Story of Blood* at http://www.pbs.org/wnet/redgold/basics/bloodgroups.html
4. Jun Hirabayashi, Faculty of Pharmaceutical Sciences: Teikyo University, Japan. www.glycoforum.gr.jp/science
5. D'Adamo, Ibid, page 187

Chapter Five Quick-Look Chart

1. For more information see: *Eat right for Your Type*, D'Adamo, Peter J. Putnam, New York, NY. 1996

Chapter Six

1. *Nutrition and Physical Degeneration*, 6th Edition, Price, Weston A., Price-Pottinger Nutrition Foundation, La Mesa, Ca. 2003. (pg. 69)

Chapter Seven

1. http://www.foodnavigator.com/news/news-NG.asp?id=44909
2. Fermented milk products would be yogurt, cottage cheese, buttermilk, and the like.

3. Reading 416-9
4. Reading 480-19
5. Reading 5097-1
6. Reading 1013-3
7. Reading 2-14
8. Reading 877-13
9. Reading 1192-6
10. Reading 5211-1
11. Reading 1852-1
12. Reading 3326-1
13. Reading 404-4
14. Reading 1158-18

Chapter 7 Food Combining Chart

1. Sometimes you are in a pinch and just cannot make an optimal food combination. In this case, go for the so-so choices. I have found that even when traveling, if you are at the mercy of what is available in any given place, you can devise a so-so combo and do all right.

2. Reading 667-8 states that "A teaspoon of [beef juice] is worth more than a quarter pound steak," likely because of the large amount of stomach acidity required to digest all that beef. In the beef juice (aka broth), you still get all the valuable amino acids and minerals.

3. The general rule is that you stay with one animal flesh per meal, unless it is the broth. Then just use common sense and don't overdo it.

4. Cayce saw milk as being taboo for some people (likely those with lactose intolerance) and excellent for others. He was much more in favor of buttermilk and yogurt "[because of the] bacilli . . . [it] will produce effects such that we will have a cleansed colon by the use of the same." (5525-1) We know now that plain organic yogurt has good benefits for the healthy intestinal flora.

5. The Cayce readings recommended stewed fruits in the morning, likely to predigest the sugars, aiding in digestion.

6. "Do not take citrus fruit juices and cereals at the same meal." (1568-2, 1484-1, etc.)

7. The good news is that cooked apples were highly recommended, "preferably roasted . . . with cinnamon and spice."

8. Yes, there are some caveats, but as a general rule, simple sugars are best when taken by themselves in small doses. This assumes there are no major health concerns. A recommendation that comes up more than once is honey mixed with heated milk "about twenty to thirty minutes before retiring [for the evening]" as helpful to counteract hypertension.

Chapter Eight

1. In other words, it is better to have yams with chicken instead of bread; carrots and/or potatoes are preferable with fish instead of rice or corn.

2. Blood Type Os will have to modify this rule just a bit to include animal proteins, just in small portions.

3. The exception here is carrots, which contain beta-carotene necessary for Level 3 people. You can mix a whole grain with carrots without any significant compromises.

4. I advise getting an informed opinion from a trusted healthcare provider prior to

purchasing any of the calcium–phosphorus–magnesium supplements in the market.

Chapter Nine
1. *Narrative of the Life of Frederick Douglass;* Bedford–St. Martin's, Boston, MA. 1993.
2. *The New Testament of the New Jerusalem Bible,* Image Books, Garden City, NY; 1986.

Chapter Ten
1. Please consult with your physician or health–care provider previous to a fast or any consequential dietary alterations, if you have a critical medical condition.
2. Although I had formulated my own anatomical measuring system via my inspiration from Traditional Chinese Medicine and Zen Shiatsu therapy, a colleague recently has directed me to the work of Jennifer Nelson, M.S., R.D., of the Mayo Clinic, where she is the director of clinical dietetics. She has presented a portion formula also based on dimensions of one's own hand. Although not identical, our two approaches are very similar. Whether it is inspiration from the same Muse or an example of "great minds think alike," I would like to acknowledge her perspective on this commonsense approach.
3. This includes high–fructose corn syrup and artificial sweeteners.
4. See recipe for vegetable juices.
5. See recipe for vegetable juices.
6. See recipe for vegetable juices.

Chapter Eleven
1. *Human Antiquity,* Fourth Edition; Feder, K.L. and Park, M.A., McGraw Hill, New York, NY. 2001
2. The Levant includes many of the countries along the Mediterranean's eastern periphery, including Egypt, Israel, Syria, Lebanon, Turkey (ancient Asia Minor), and Greece.
3. http://www.usda.gov/factbook/chapter2.htm
4. http://www.imdb.com/title/tt0062622/quotes

Chapter Twelve
1. Portions excerpted from http://www.foodreference.com/html/html/yearonlytimeline.html, and http://www.gti.net/mocolib1/kid/food.html
2. http://www.hort.purdue.edu/newcrop/proceedings1996/V3-479.html#HISTORY; Heiser, C.B. 1976. Peppers Capsicum (Solanaceae). p. 265–268. In: N.W. Simmonds (ed.), The evolution of crops plants. Longman Press, London; Heiser, C.B. and P.G. Smith. 1953. The cultivated Capsicum peppers. Econ. Bot. 7:214–227; MacNeish, R.S. 1964. Ancient Mesoamerican civilization. Science 143:531–537.
3. http://www.hort.purdue.edu/newcrop/morton/citron.html
4. http://www.internationaloliveoil.org/tm/usa/about_history.asp
5. http://www.hort.wisc.edu/usdavcru/simon/garlic_origins.html
6. http://www.meccagold.com/history.htm
7. http://webexhibits.org/butter/
8. http://www.botgard.ucla.edu/html/botanytextbooks/economicbotany/Ceratonia/index.html
9. http://www.horseradish.org/history.html
10. *UCLA History and Special Collections,* Louise M. Darling Biomedical Library; http://unitproj.library.ucla.edu/biomed/spice/index.cfm?displayID=5
11. http://aggie-horticulture.tamu.edu/plantanswers/publications/vegetabletravelers/beets.html

12. *The Cambridge World History of Food*, II.D.1; http://www.cup.org/books/kiple/chestnuts.htm

13. Social Issues Research Center; http://www.sirc.org/timeline/55.shtml, Whelan, E.M. & Stare, F.J. (1992) *Panic in the Pantry*. Prometheus Books, Amherst, NY. [with thanks to Stephen Barrett, MD.]

14. http://www.sirc.org/timeline/123.shtml ;Lieberman, L.S. (2000) *Diet and Chronic Disease*. Cambridge World History of Food. Cambridge University Press.

15. Social Issues Research Center; http://www.sirc.org/timeline/170.shtml; Grivetti, L.E. (2000) *Food Prejudices and Taboos*. Cambridge World History of Food. Cambridge University Press.

16. http://www.sushiman.net/sushi/history.htm

17. Social Issues Research Center; http://www.sirc.org/timeline/400.shtml; Grivetti, L.E. (2000) *Food Prejudices and Taboos*. Cambridge World History of Food. Cambridge University Press.

18. http://aggie-horticulture.tamu.edu/plantanswers/publications/vegetabletravelers/peas.html

19. http://www.nationalgeographic.com/coffee/ax/frame.html

20. Social Issues Research Center; http://www.sirc.org/timeline/1200.shtml; Grivetti, L.E. (2000) *Food Prejudices and Taboos*. Cambridge World History of Food. Cambridge University Press.

21. Social Issues Research Center; http://www.sirc.org/timeline/1500.shtml

22. http://www.siu.edu/~ebl/leaflets/tomato.htm

23. http://www.sirc.org/timeline/1550.shtml; Whorton, J. (1982) Crusaders for fitness: the history of American health reformers. Princeton University Press. USA

24. http://www.sirc.org/timeline/1734.shtml

25. Some sources cite *American Cookery*, published in 1776 as the first American cookbook.

26. http://www.sirc.org/timeline/1790.shtml;Harper, A.E. (2000) *Recommended Dietary Allowances and Dietary Guidance*. Cambridge World History of Food. Cambridge University Press.

27. http://www.sirc.org/timeline/1848.shtml; Whelan, E.M. & Stare, F.J. (1992) *Panic in the Pantry*. Prometheus Books, Amherst, NY. [with thanks to Stephen Barrett, MD.]

28. http://www.sirc.org/timeline/1800.shtml; Beard, G. (1871) *Eating and Drinking*. New York. USA. cited in Brumberg, J.J. (1988) *Fasting Girls; The Emergence of Anorexia Nervosa as a Modern Disease*. Harvard University Press. USA.

29. FDA Backgrounder; http://vm.cfsan.fda.gov/mileston.html

30. http://www.sirc.org/timeline/1885.shtml; Levenstein H.A. (1988) *Revolution at the Table: The Transformation of the American Diet*, Oxford University Press, New York, 1993.

31. http://www.sirc.org/timeline/1902.shtml

32. http://www.sirc.org/timeline/1911.shtml ; Whelan, E.M. & Stare, F.J. (1992) *Panic in the Pantry*. Prometheus Books, Amherst, NY. [with thanks to Stephen Barrett, MD.]

33. http://www.sirc.org/timeline/1950.shtml; Gofman, J W, et al. The role of lipids and lipoproteins in arteriosclerosis. Science 1950; 111: 166–181, 186

34. FDA Backgrounder

35. http://www.sirc.org/timeline/1960.shtml; Coveney, J. (2000) *Food, Morals and Meaning. The Pleasure and Anxiety of Eating*. Routledge.

36. "FDA officials said that, since 1981, about 8,000 consumers have complained to the agency that the sweetener has caused them physical ailments, including headaches, nausea, vision problems, and seizures. Scientists consider such reports anecdotal and not proof of a causal relationship.

[Toxicologist James] Huff said that the number of reports is worrisome, though, because "if 100 people have a headache after chewing NutraSweet gum, only one's going to report it." http://users.westnet.gr/~cgian/fda1.htm

37. http://www.sirc.org/timeline/1985.shtml; Coveney, J. (2000) *Food, Morals and Meaning. The Pleasure and Anxiety of Eating.* Routledge.

38. Controversies abound over the safety of this product. According to a study conducted by Health Canada, the cows treated with rBST had "approximately a 25% increase in the risk of clinical mastitis ... a number of effects on reproductive performance ... approximately a 50% increase in the risk of clinical lameness ... " and "the panel concluded that the use of rBST would likely reduce the lifespan of dairy cattle." www.hc-sc.gc.ca/english/protection/rbst/animals/14.htm

39. BBC News, Monday, March 31st, 2003; http://news.bbc.co.uk/1/hi/health/2903739.stm

Chapter Fourteen

1. http://cancerweb.ncl.ac.uk/cancernet/600037.html

2. According to the U.S. Census Bureau, Jan. 1, 2005. www.census.gov

3. Tuormaa, Tuula E., FORESIGHT, the Association for the Promotion of Preconceptual Care; published in Journal of Orthomolecular Medicine, 9(4): 225–243, 1994.

4. Egger J, Carter CM, Graham PJ, Gumley D, Soothill JF: Controlled Trial of Oligoantigenic Treatment in the Hyperkinetic Syndrome. The Lancet, 540–545, March 9, 1985.

5. Miller M and Millstone E: *Food Additives Campaign Team: Report on Colour Additives.* FACT, 25 Horsell Road, London N5 1XL, June, 1987.

6. Schauss AG: Nutrition and Behavior: Complex Interdisciplinary Research. Nutrition and Health, 3:9–37, 1984 and Bryce–Smith D: Environmental and Chemical Influences on Behavior and Mentation. (John Leyes Lecture) Chem Soc Rev, 15:93–123, 1986

7. http://www.westonaprice.org/motherlinda/cornsyrup.html

8. PR Web, http://www.prweb.com/releases/2004/8/prweb145651.htm

9. Journal of the American College of Nutrition, Vol. 17, No. 4, 317–321 (1998), http://www.jacn.org/cgi/content/full/17/4/317

Chapter Fifteen

1. Better Homes and Gardens, July 1998; David Feder; http://articles.findarticles.com/p/articles/mi_m1041/is_n7_v76/ai_20806523

2. Iatrogenic means that it is unintentionally caused by the physician, surgeon, treatment plan, or diagnostic procedure. In other words, the person or plan that is supposed to cure you, injures you.

3. The 1998 study estimated that 106,000 people a year die as a result of an adverse reaction to a prescription medication. This statistic reflects medicines taken exactly as directed and does not include intentional overdosing. (J Lazarou, B.M. Pomeranz, P.N. Corey, Journal of the American Medical Association, Apr. 15, 1998; 279:1200–5.)

4. Specific national statistics on surgery mishaps are very difficult to obtain since there is no medical coding for "surgical mistake;" the business of medicine has too few systems for accurately calculating its own ineffectiveness. Researchers know that there are problems that need addressing. In an October 8, 2003, JAMA study from the Federal government's Agency for Healthcare Research and Quality (AHRQ), 32,000 primarily surgery–related deaths were studied. Among the incidents analyzed: post-

operative bleeding, surgical wounds reopening, foreign objects left in wounds, and post–operative infections.

5. http://www.foodnavigator.com/news/news-NG.asp?id=9155
6. http://www.mercola.com/2003/dec/13/holiday_spices.htm
7. http://www.confex.com/ift/99annual/abstracts/4254.htm
8. There are actually about 26,000, based on some estimates. It is theorized that there are approximately a quarter of a million plants identified as having the potential for medicinal benefits, but these have not been fully researched. This does not account for the tens, perhaps hundreds, of thousands of plant and fungi varieties that have yet to be discovered. Nature is indeed replete with wisdom and usefulness.
9. Ishikawa, K., R. Naganawa, H. Yoshida, N. Iwata, H. Fukuda, T. Fujino, and A. Suzuki. 1996. Antimutagenic Effects of Ajoene, an Arganosulfur Compound Derived from Garlic. Bioscience, Biotechnology, and Biochemistry 60: 2086–2088.
Ishikawa, K., R. Naganawa, H. Yoshida, N. Iwata, H. Fukuda, T. Fujino, and A. Suzuki. 1996. Inhibition of Microbial Growth by Ajoene, a Sulfur Compound Derived from Garlic. Applied and Environmental Microbiology 62: 4238–4243.
Davis, D.L. 1989. Natural Anticarcinogens, Carcinogens, and Changing Patterns in Cancer: Some Speculation. Environmental Research 50: 322–340.
10. Boyle, W. 1991. *Official Herbs: Botanical Substances in the United States Pharmacopoeias 1820-1990.* East Palestine, OH: Buckeye Naturopathic Press.

Chapter Sixteen
1. Ambergris is a gray substance found in the intestine of the sperm whale. When heated, it emits a perfume of sorts. It was apparently found floating on top of the waters near coasts of warm climate countries. Since 1977, the U.S. has banned the use of whale products in the commercial marketplace (see notes to reading 953-1).

A.R.E. PRESS

The A.R.E. Press publishes books, videos, and audiotapes meant to improve the quality of our readers' lives—personally, professionally, and spiritually. We hope our products support your endeavors to realize your career potential, to enhance your relationships, to improve your health, and to encourage you to make the changes necessary to live a loving, joyful, and fulfilling life.

For more information or to receive a free catalog, call:

1–800–723–1112

Or write:

A.R.E. Press
215 67th Street
Virginia Beach, VA 23451-2061

BAAR PRODUCTS

A.R.E.'s Official Worldwide Exclusive Supplier of Edgar Cayce Health Care Products

Baar Products, Inc., is the official worldwide exclusive supplier of Edgar Cayce health care products. Baar offers a collection of natural products and remedies drawn from the work of Edgar Cayce, considered by many to be the father of modern holistic medicine.

For a complete listing of Cayce-related products, call:

1–800–269–2502

Or write:

Baar Products, Inc.
P.O. Box 60
Downingtown, PA 19335 U.S.A.

Customer Service and International: 610–873–4591
Fax: 610–873–7945
Web Site: www.baar.com   E-mail: cayce@baar.com